HUALMA,

THE PERUVIAN.

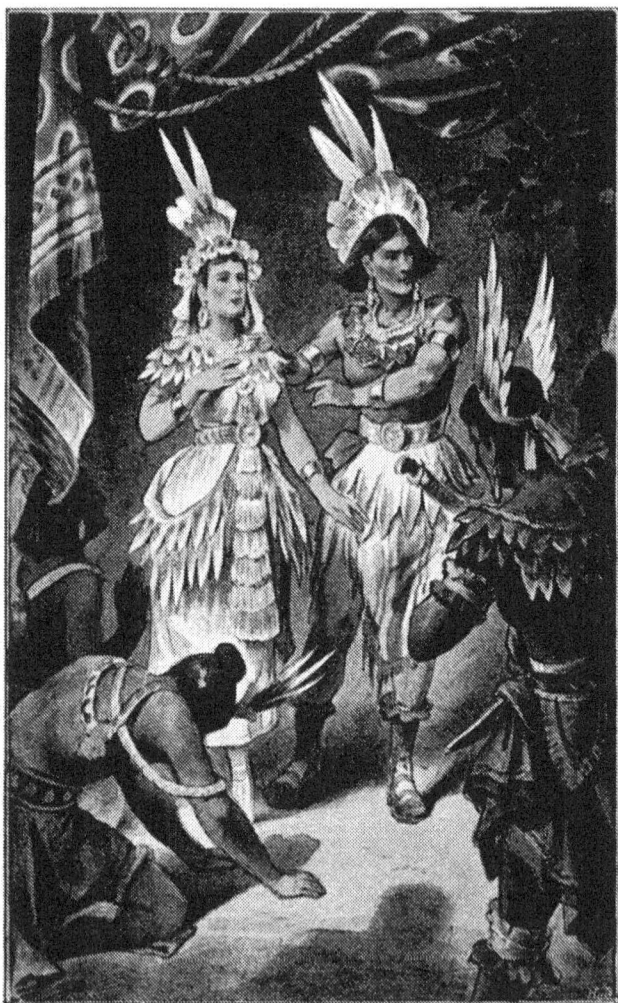

HUALMA,

THE PERUVIAN.

THE STORY OF THE DISCOVERY OF QUININE

BY

W. O. von HORN.

TRANSLATED FROM THE GERMAN.

Fredonia Books
Amsterdam, The Netherlands

Hualma, The Peruvian:
The Story of the Discovery of Quinine

by
W. O. von Horn

ISBN: 1-4101-0269-6

Fredonia Books
Amsterdam, The Netherlands
http://www.fredoniabooks.com

CHAPTER I.

The virey, Count Fernando Cinchon, had now been two years in Lima. Virey is an abbreviation of viceroy, and was the official title of the representative of the king of Spain. His treatment of the inhabitants of the city and of the Indians of the Cordillera de los Andes, that is the mighty mountain range of Peru, had been such, that for a long time there had been no breach of peace between the Indians and the Spaniards. He hoped that the friendly relations would not again be broken, and that the country for a long time to come would enjoy the benefits of peace. If all Spaniards had been like him, his fond hope might have been realized. Unfortunately however, the oppression and abuse of the Indians was not stopped, even under his mild rule, and without his knowledge, the clouds were beginning to gather thickly in consequence.

It was in the year 1556 when he received word, that his only child, his young daughter Dolores, who had been educated in a convent in Spain, was on her way to join him. She was all he had, for his dear wife had fallen sick on the voyage from Palos in Spain to Lima, and had died in Callao shortly after landing.

He had spent the dreariest period of his life in Lima, where he had no one with whom he could intimately associate. But now the future began to look brighter. Dolores was coming to cheer his days, to drive away his cares, to fill his heart with gladness, and to bring joy into the lonely, monotonous life at Lima. It was indeed a happy prospect for this man, who was susceptible of every good impression, who honestly and faithfully strove for the right, and in the line of the viceroys of Peru, made a notable exception. All thoughts of a war with the Indians, which threatened to break out sooner or later, were crowded into the back-ground with all their fears and anxieties. He gave himself fully over to a foretaste of the joy of a father's heart at the coming of his child. It was his intention on the following morning to go to Callao, there to await her coming.

After a very hot day there had come a cool, refreshing evening. The count stepped out on the balcony of the palace, where he resided, in order to enjoy the air. This balcony overlooked a large square, in which frequently thousands promenaded. The square was surrounded by large buildings, among these the fine cathedral. But to-night the place was almost empty, and dull quiet lay over it, while at other times it was filled with the hum of many voices. This seemed strange to him and somewhat troubled him. Perhaps the fickle citizens, he told himself, had gone to the boulevard before the gate of Callao. Just then the draught from the room, in front of which was the balcony, told him that the door had been opened. A negro appeared and announced the chief magistrate of Lima.

The virey entered the room and found there awaiting him, a tall, rather slender Spaniard clothed in black. In spite of the warm weather he wore a mantle, and in his hand he held a hat adorned with a long, waving feather. About his neck he wore a large, white ruffled collar, and from a heavy golden chain, there hung upon his breast, a large golden medallion, the symbol of his office.

Don Cinchon looked sharply into his thin, yellow face, and into his large black eyes, which lay deep in their sockets. The expression of his face and the look in his eyes promised no good news from the lips of the magistrate.

"If I rightly interpret the expression of your face,"

said the virey not without an anxious presentiment, "you are the bearer of bad news."

"Unfortunately," answered the magistrate bowing low.

"Gracious lord," the magistrate continued, "it is doubly sad news."

"How so?" quickly asked Count Cinchon.

"On the one hand we shall have war with the Indians, on the other hand we have to expect a famine in Lima."

The virey grew pale, but he remained silent as if he expected further details.

The magistrate well understood his questioning silence and continued: "For two days no Indian has appeared upon the market-place, and your lordship knows, that we have to depend upon the Indians for our provisions. They bring feed for our horses and mules, and this being cut off the animals must die. Moreover without their supply of meat and excellent fruits we shall starve. They are the only source from which we draw our means of subsistence."

"Well," said Cinchon, "you speak to me of things of which I have no knowledge whatever."

"I can well understand that," replied the magistrate, "but I know all the more about them, because it is my duty to watch the public market, where our citizens satisfy their wants."

"But why has not care been taken in Lima to secure the absolute necessities of life, in such cases, in towns lying nearer the coast?" asked Cinchon.

"Gracious lord," replied the magistrate, "that might be possible during the rainy season, but during the hot months even the low country must draw supplies from the mountains. During this season vegetation dies down there, and the country is practically a desert."

The virey made a troubled face. "But what is to be done?" he asked in great perplexity.

"We can be saved only by a quick attack upon the Indians," answered the magistrate with great earnestness.

"But we are not at all clear as to the intentions of the Indians," said Count Cinchon.

Before the magistrate could answer, the negro again entered to announce Father Escobar of the Jesuit mission "El Ingenio", who begged for instant audience, as he had a most important matter to communicate.

"Your lordship will learn more from him than I can tell," said the magistrate, as he bowed and retired a few paces.

At the same time the door opened, and there entered a middle aged man of imposing appearance. A bandage was bound about his head, and his coat hung in rags. His face was pale, and he was scarcely able to keep himself on his feet.

The virey hastened toward him, took him respectfully by the hand, and led him to a chair, where he sank down.

"Forgive me, kind sir," said he feebly, "that I come to you in such a state. My mule, speedy as the wind, saved me when the Indians took our beautiful mission and burned it to the ground. They pursued me to the very gates of the city. A turn of my head saved me from being killed by the tomahawk, which caused this wound. When I reached the first houses of Lima, I fell fainting from my mule, and some good soul took pity on me, and bound up my wound. Brother Ambrosio is dead, the hacienda is levelled to the ground, and our magnificent sugar plantation is devastated. Our blacks and superintendents were all murdered. You see me before you a beggar."

"My God!" cried the virey, "and all this comes so suddenly?"

"No," said Father Escobar, "it was planned in secret, and preparations have been making for a long time, but no one had any suspicion until now."

"I knew of nothing," cried Cinchon.

"That is the way of these devils," cried the priest, trembling with rage. "They lay their plans in deepest secresy and when everything is ready, they break out in wildest cruelty, like a mountain stream, swollen by a cloudburst. This is the reason they strike so heavy and so sure, because no one has any suspicion, and no precautions have been taken."

"Are you acquainted with any details of the case, reverend father?" asked Cinchon.

Escobar recounted, that a descendant of the reigning family of the Incas had escaped, and lived in the distant mountains of Chili. His name was Huahamac. He was distinguished before all by the shrewdness with which he took advantage of opportunities, by his burning hatred of the whites and his extraordinary bravery. All the mountain tribes were under his command, and this time it would be a struggle for life or death, of annihilation of the Spaniards or the Indians. They were encamped between the mission "El Ingenio" and Lima. A few days would suffice to attack Lima, and destroy it, unless measures of defence were at once taken.

This was the substance of a long, exhaustive explanation, which the virey however, followed with closest attention.

It was now his duty to take the necessary steps to defend the city. He dismissed the magistrate and the jesuit, and then summoned the officers of his soldiers, with whom he held a council of war.

This council lasted until far into the night. In the meantime a special messenger from the commandant at Callao brought him word, that the vessel on which his daughter had taken passage, lay at anchor in the harbor. The young lady wished to land on the following morning, in order to hasten to him.

He informed his council of this circumstance, and declared at the same time, that he would himself go to meet his daughter. For this reason he appointed an old experienced general to act in his stead during his absence.

No one tried to dissuade him from his plan, but all strongly urged him to take along an escort of one hundred cavalry. The Indians seemed to be kept perfectly informed about everything transpiring in the city, and the virey in going or returning, might easily fall into an ambush.

Every man was assigned his particular duty, every man was appointed to his special post, and only after all this had been arranged, was an adjutant dispatched to select the escort for the virey, which was to be ready early the following morning.

The night, in which an attack of the redskins might be expected, and for which they had carefully prepared themselves, passed quietly enough. Not however, for the virey. He could not sleep, nevertheless he was up bright and early in the morning. Arming himself completely, he mounted his battle-horse. One hundred tried and trusty horsemen joined him. The day had scarely dawned, when they rode down the broad main avenue of the city, and passing through the gate, followed the road toward Callao. A slight mist hung over the landscape, but as the sun came up, it disappeared quickly.

The road they were following, was the popular promenade of the Limennos, as the inhabitants of Lima are called, and therefore bore the name Alameda de Callao. To the right of it there stretched away the lowlands, overgrown with rushes and reed-grass, to the banks of the Rimac river, which divides Lima into two unequal parts. The low mounds in this part of the country appeared as perfectly bare sand-hills. The view was wretched. Even the rushes and reed-grass had succumbed to the heat, and appeared burned and yellow. To the left the country gradually rose to a moderate height, crowned with woods. The sides of the mountain were here thickly covered with brushwood as far as the Alameda de Callao.

A profound silence lay upon the scene. There were few animals in that region, and even birds were scarce, excepting the vultures, which fill the position of scavengers, keeping clean the roads and streets, upon which the people carelessly threw any refuse matter. They were seen now, flying toward the city from all directions, in search of their morning meal.

At Cinchon's side rode old Don Perez, a warrior of great experience, who had grown gray in the service in Peru. His keen eyes sharply scanned the brushwood at the side of the road. Even when he answered the few questions which Cinchon addressed to him, he kept his face turned toward the side of the road. The virey noticed this and finally asked of him the reason for his peculiar action.

"We shall probably very soon find out the good reason for my looking in that direction," said he. "I must have been very much mistaken, if I did not a little while ago, see the head of a redskin, who was watching our approach. Lances up and tinder in readiness!" he thundered to the horsemen. The virey looked at him in astonishment, while the horsemen instantly obeyed the order.

"What is the meaning of this?" he quickly asked.

"Here is the answer," cried the commander. A cloud of arrows whizzed through the air. Instantly it seemed as if several Indians rose out of every bush. Their war-whoop was the most horrible sound which had ever entered Cinchon's ear.

It was fortunate for the Spaniards, that the arrows had been shot from such a distance as to make them ineffective. The command of their leader caused the troop to wheel about instantly, and in swift gallop they threw themselves upon the enemy. The Indians feared two things with the Spaniards, their long spears, which became dangerous from a considerable distance, and their firearms. They seldom held out over against these two, especially if their arrows rebounded harmlessly from the iron armor of the Spaniards. This was a wellknown fact.

The red-skins had been carefully watching the Spaniards, but the sharp eye of Don Perez had detected them, and he had compelled them to shoot sooner than was their intention. Thus it came, that to their dismay, they saw that their arrows did not reach their goal. The swift attack of the Spaniards was more stubbornly resisted by them than ever before in the experience of that old fighter, Don Perez. Swinging their tomahawks, they rushed out from behind their cover, and sprang forward to battle. But thereby they exposed their naked bodies to the enemy. The Spaniards took careful aim and fired. The Indians fell like snow-flakes; but this did not keep them from renewing the attack with the greatest fury. Since there was no time to reload, the Spaniards brought their spears into action. Again they had a decided advantage. Although in other battles the Indians had always taken to flight before this weapon, the situation had changed now. With the greatest bravery they pressed forward, and the battle became hotter and fiercer than ever. More and more it became a single combat between the Spaniards and the Indians, who were their superiors in numbers. The swords were torn from their scabbards, and soon again the Spaniards found the advantage on their side. Still the result of the battle might have remained doubtful, if a cloud of dust moving rapidly along the Alameda de Callao, had not told the Indians, that a new danger was threatening them by the approach of re-enforcements for the Spaniards. Don Perez, foreseeing an ambuscade, had arranged for these, and by good fortune, they arrived upon the scene of battle in the nick of time.

Count Cinchon, ever brave in fight, had remained by the side of Don Perez, until the irregular battle, caused by the underbrush, had separated them. A gigantic chief hurled himself against him. The color of this Indian's skin was somewhat lighter than that of the other savages. His ornaments also distinguished him. From his head there waved a crown of feathers, such as none of the other Indians wore. He fell upon the count with terrible fury. The blows of his tomahawk hailed upon him, and in spite of his agility in battle, Count Cinchon would not have been able long to withstand him, had it not been for his excellent armor and trusty shield. The Indian was already bleeding from several wounds, which gave him a most horrible appearance. Just as five Indians were rushing to the aid of their chief, Don Perez, who had struck down an Indian but a moment before, discovered the perilous position of the virey, and hastened to his assistance. One powerful sidelong blow dealt by Don Perez stretched the chief to earth. The other Indians, who now also discovered the flight of their comrades before the Spaniards, swiftly sped away. The Spaniards pursued the fleeing Indians far up the mountain side, covering the ground with wounded and slain. But the flight of the Indians was far too swift, so that the Spaniards, because the ground was unsuited for cavalry fighting, could not completely wipe them out.

A half hour later no enemy was anywhere to be seen. The battlefield covered with the bodies of the wounded and the slain, showed how awful had been the defeat of the Indians.

But now there began a slaughter, which the noble Don Cinchon tried in vain to prevent. Like cruel tigers the Spaniards drove their spears into the hearts of the wounded, until there breathed not one of them. It was only the great influence of the virey, and his threat to strike down anyone who raised a hand against him, that saved the chief from certain death under the very eyes of Cinchon.

The chief had received several very deep cuts. His head bore particularly severe wounds.

Cinchon dismounted, in order to examine his wounds.

"Don't you worry about him," said Don Perez, "such an Indian skull is thick and hard. It is true, he is very badly cut up, but I will wager my sword against his tomahawk, that he will come to and be healed before you imagine. They have a life as tenacious as that of a cat."

A soldier who knew about the application of bandages was called, and at the express command of the virey, bound up the wounds of the chief.

"Do you notice the golden sun on his breast?" cried Perez. "If this be not the Inca Huahamac himself, whom you have brought down, I must be very much mistaken indeed."

"Would to God it were true!" said Don Cinchon, as he looked upon his stricken foe with deep sympathy and pity. "There would be hope of the speedy reestablishment of peace."

"True," returned Perez; "for the serpent would have lost its head. But mark you, I have no inclination to make light of the lashings of the tail. However, our enemies have suffered a heavy defeat, and for a few days at least, Lima is safe from them. I doubt whether it will be for a longer time, since I know well the nature of these redskins."

While this conversation was going on the chief had been skilfully bound up. Water had been carefully given him to drink, and from the canteen of one of the soldiers, he had been bathed with it. Under these applications he at last opened his eyes. Quickly he raised his gigantic body to a sitting posture. He cast one swift glance over the battlefield, and as the certainty of a complete victory by the Spaniards came to him, he quickly tore a daggerlike knife from his belt, in order to plunge it into his heart. But Don Perez had been narrowly watching him, and with an iron grasp now seized and held his hand. The knife fell from his fingers and Don Perez picked it up. Then the Indian began to tear off his bandages. Only after he had been securely bound with ropes, and rendered perfectly helpless, could he be prevented from carrying out his purpose of escaping captivity by committing suicide.

Several hours passed while the things which have been related were happening. Men and horses stood in need of rest, in order to continue the journey to Callao under the scorching rays of the sun. The old willows which lined the road, offered scarcely enough protection. The sun burned down upon them, and the iron armor of the Spaniards became hot to suffocation. Prudence however, commanded to remain in armor in order to be prepared for an attack. It was possible that the Indians would make an effort to rescue their captured Inca.

With great difficulty Don Cinchon restrained his eagerness to press to his heart his darling child, the last and dearest treasure of his life. He was not at all tired, although he had fought with great bravery at the head of his company. He recognized the necessity however, of giving rest to both men and horses. He would have gone on to Callao alone, for it was but a few miles distant, but his escort would not permit it.

At last they started off. Now Perez was extraordinarily happy. The victory had been easily won. Only three of his men had been wounded, and these so slightly, that they were not even prevented from accompanying their honored virey to Callao.

But the most important circumstance was the capture of Huahamac, the Inca. Perez did not for one instant doubt that the captured chief was the very soul and spirit of the uprising of the Indians. The captive was turned over to the leader of the troops, who had come from Lima to reenforce them. Cinchon impressed it upon him, that he would be held personally responsible for any harm which might be inflicted upon the chief, who was to be kept in the virey's palace, and treated very kindly. Then they parted. The troops returned to Lima, while Cinchon and Perez together with their escort, accompanied the litter, borne by carefully chosen mules. On they went toward the shore of the ocean, which soon lay before them in all its immeasurable expanse, its deep blue waters smooth as glass in a perfect calm.

Cinchon's thoughts were with his child, awaiting him in the city far below them. He was only half attentive to the enthusiastic stories Don Perez was telling him of his experience as an Indian fighter. Yet though he did not give him his full attention, Cinchon frequently shuddered when he heard of the wild barbarities, which Perez praised as deeds of valor. Such speeches, like the deeds which they described, showed how inhumanly a harmless people was being treated. Men seemed actually to consider it a good work to slaughter the natives. Yet the fruit of such a sowing could not but be irreconcilable, mortal hatred of the whites by the Indians, who had been made so wretched. Now the towers of Callao appeared. They saw the shipping in the harbor, and from the flagstaff on the house of the port-officer they saw waving the great flag, which showed that Donna Dolores, the daughter of the powerful virey of Peru, was stopping there.

The ground began to gently slope toward the coast, and giving the reins to his horse, the virey sped forward. Behind him followed the escort, still bearing the traces of the bloody work they had but just done, in the blood-stains on their armor. A few minutes later, the lady, weeping tears of joy, lay upon her happy father's bosom.

Cinchon could not weary of gazing upon her. During the time he had been compelled to leave her in Spain, she had ripened into womanhood, lovely as the opening rose, the faithful image of her mother. The happiness of the father knew no bounds, and even the stony hearts of the soldiers were moved, as they witnessed the happiness and joy of father and child. For, breaking through the formality of strict old Spanish etiquette and custom, these two followed the natural promptings of their hearts in their first greeting.

Both riders and horses took a good rest in Callao. The men were richly entertained, and the horses were well fed, having had but small rations in the morning, on account of the lack of fodder in consequence of the Indian uprising.

The conditions in Lima, and the fight with the Indians, did not permit of more than a few hours rest. Perez only waited for the time, when the day being spent, it began to grow cooler, and then in a modest way reminded the virey that the time for the return had arrived.

Cinchon could not refrain from asking the question, whether another attack by the Indians was to be feared on the return. Perez knew very well that he asked this, on account of his daughter.

"Most certainly not," said Perez. "They have already withdrawn far into the mountains. I only feared a second attack while they were yet in the neighbourhood, and because their chief was in our hands, and finally because they were not likely to leave their dead in our power, or at the mercy of the vultures. Their customs forbid that. But their retreat is explained in the same way. With the bodies of their dead they are hurrying away to a safe distance. We shall be secure from any attack while they are performing their rights over the dead, unless we seek them out ourselves, a thing I strongly recommend. Another defeat will take away the last bit of their courage, and compel them to sue for peace. The unfortunate condition of things in Lima, as well as the desire to prevent years of hostilities, urge this upon us. The longer a war with them lasts, the more serious it grows for us."

The virey thoughtfully listened to this well considered advice. He compared it with what had been communicated to him by the magistrate of Lima and Father Escobar, and its truth became as clear as day to his mind. He therefore urged a speedy departure, and soon the company was ready. Donna Dolores and her "duenna", or governess and companion, an elderly lady, entered the litter, whose mules were led by negroes dressed in rich livery. Her maids rode behind the splendidly ornamented litter on gorgeously caparrisoned mules. To the right of the litter her father took his place, while Don Perez rode on the left. The escort took the litter in their midst. The company having thus been formed, they left Callao.

Cinchon gave himself up to the full enjoyment of

his daughter's company. She had so much to tell him about his country, his old friends and the different members of the distinguished and wealthy family of Cinchon, that he found no time to think of anything else. But old Don Perez gave all the more heed to those things required for their safety.

Although many years full of experience had passed over him, he appeared almost youthful in bearing and action. His eye was as keen as that of the condor, the mighty bird of the Andes mountains, which from dizzy heights spies its prey amid the low shrubbery. Perez paid no attention to things near him, but the brush-covered hills lying to the right, and rising toward the thickly wooded highlands, these he sharply searched. No branch moved in the wind, but he keenly looked to see whether anything suspicious showed itself. From long experience he well knew the trickiness and treachery of the enemy. He knew how they could in the most marvellous manner cover themselves, until the moment favorable to them arrived and was instantly used. For this reason he not only noted every moving twig, but every sound, every call of bird or beast, he carefully observed, for these might well have been the signals of a hidden foe.

This time however, there was no danger. There appeared no sign of trouble anywhere. When they came near to the place where the dreadful, bloody work had been done, and saw no trace of a dead body, the last care departed from his soul, and he gave his attention to other matters.

The officer who had carried the flag furled up, since the little company had left Lima, now received the order to unfurl it. This was a signal which had been agreed upon. As soon as the flag was seen waving in the breeze, all the church-bells in Lima began to ring. At the same time a procession emerged from the city gates, and approached them on the Alameda. Crowds of young girls dressed in white and carrying palms, headed the procession. They were followed by the priests of the city, clothed in their magnificent robes. After these came the city officials, soldiers and citizens.

The honor was shown not so much to the daughter of the virey, as rather to Don Cinchon himself. The city took this occasion to show how highly it respected and loved him.

There were costly gifts presented to the young lady, addresses were delivered, and incense burned by the priests. The archbishop of Lima gave his benediction at the close of the celebration. Then the procession was again formed, all the riders following the litter.

Thus they moved along between dense crowds of people, who shouted themselves hoarse in joyous greeting, until they arrived at the Plaza Major, as the great square in front of the virey's palace was called.

The virey himself assisted his beautiful daughter to alight from her litter. Taking her by the hand he led her into the cathedral, where a service was held, to implore God's blessing for the young lady and to render praise and thanksgiving for the victory which had been won. After the religious ceremonies the virey brought his daughter to the palace, a plain, though massive structure, which Pizarro, the conqueror of Peru, had built.

While she was comfortably settling herself in her new home, Don Cinchon presided at a council of war. Perez gave it as his opinion, that the small, yet strong army should set out very early on the following morning, to seek out the Indians in their hiding places. This plan prevailed.

While Cinchon was loath thus to leave his daughter,

when she had scarcely entered his home, he was nevertheless much comforted by the assurance of Father Escobar, that his prisoner really was Huahamac, a descendant of the powerful family of Incas, who had once ruled over the land. The head of the rebellious Indians was in his hands, and under the circumstances, was doing very well.

Cinchon had a hard struggle against the demands raised on all sides, that Huahamac be burned at the stake according to an old Spanish custom. However, his will was law, although his view, that Christian charity must at last take the place of harshness and brutality, was not accepted by these hard-hearted, cruel men.

That very night he visited his prisoner, and to his satisfaction he found him much more resigned to his fate. The care which he received did him good, and when the noble virey visited him in his prison cell, and assured him of a mild and gentle treatment, that broke his pride, and he felt his heart swell with a feeling which he had thought he could never entertain for any Spaniard. Cinchon did more. He commended the wounded prisoner to the care of his daughter, when he found that he would have to leave Lima for a time.

CHAPTER II.

It was a sore trial for Dolores, that she had to be separated from her dear father so soon after her arrival. She bore it the more heavily because he was going out to battle, and would be exposed to the greatest dangers. Don Cinchon pressed the weeping girl to his bosom, and sought to comfort her. He told her to put her whole trust in Him who alone can give sure protection and safety.

"Pray for me, dear Dolores," said he; "and God will give His angels charge over me, to keep me in safety. — One thing more. Be gentle with our prisoner. You can not speak with him, but everybody understands deeds of kindness, even though he may not be able to understand words of kindness, which are spoken to him. Deeds of kindness are acceptable to God. May He keep you. I know that you will do what I have asked of you."

Then he hastened away, mounted his steed, and disappeared down the street, which led through the city gate to the mountains. The troops were already assembled, and they set out at once.

The men were well equipped, and courage filled their hearts and souls. And there was need of careful equipment and a stout heart, for the marches were long and frequently those in the van had to make a road for those who followed. When night came they sank down utterly worn out, to sleep under the open sky. The intense heat also wearied them very much. It was a fortunate thing that there was no lack of delicious, nourishing fruits, and that there was an abundance of fine clear springs. Besides they were in the very home of that plant which we praise as one of God's best gifts to man, the potato. Sir Frances Drake first brought it to England in 1586, and since then it has come to be one of the most indispensable articles of food. The season of its full growth was here, and they thus found everywhere the most wholesome and nourishing food. They prepared the potatoes by roasting them in the fire.

Don Perez had sent ahead as scouts two negroes, who had served him well in the previous Indian war. They returned on the evening of the third day, and noiselessly slipped into the old fighter's tent. They reported that they had found the Indians engaged in their funeral rites in a deep valley, only a few hours'march distant. The Indians seemed to have no idea that their enemies were so near. The scouts had even found the very best routes, by which it would be possible to attack the Indians from two sides at once.

Now Perez was sure of his undertaking. When the day broke he communicated to the virey what his scouts had reported. Then he divided his troops into two equal companies, and appointed one of the negroes for each to act as guide. · He took the leadership of that troop which was to attack the enemy from behind, because the virey desired to head the company which was to make the direct attack.

Everything had been carefully considered in the council of war. And so they set out on that march which at last was to bring them face to face with the foe. Victory was certain, and yet Cinchon was not glad, was not happy.

The route led through narrow passes, and then to a shallow creek whose course they followed. It led them straight into the valley where the Indians were encamped. Now they had to make haste to get out of the narrow gorge before the Indians could learn of their approach.

It was almost incredible when one considers the great shrewdness of the Indians, that they should have had no warning of the coming of their foes. Yet this was the case, and so secure did they feel themselves, that they had made no provisions whatever for their safety. They depended upon the exceptional seclusion of this valley in which they were encamped.

Their terror was indescribable when the horsemen

suddenly broke from the forest which surrounded the valley, and when they saw the musketeers advance upon them. Thousands of them, for their numbers were great, hurled themselves against the foe. Thousands of them turned to flee into the forests, but Don Perez awaited them here, and there began a fearful massacre. Most of them turned back and brought confusion into the ranks of those who had courageously thrown themselves against the troops led by Don Cinchon.

And now Don Perez and his troops broke forth from the forest, and there began a slaughter which we would rather not describe. The heart shudders at its very thought. Even to this day that valley in the heart of the Cordillera de los Andes, two days journey from Lima. is known as the "Valley of Blood".

It could truthfully be said, that the army of Huahamac was annihilated, the insurrection quelled in its very beginning, and the power of the Indians broken for a long time to come. And even though many of them escaped from the battle, or rather massacre, that made no difference in the result. The capture of their chief had already been of most discouraging influence. They clung to him with touching fidelity, and his loss left them without an adviser and leader. Their courage was broken, and now there came this terrible defeat to show them how utterly their plan to secure absolute liberty had failed.

Two days later they sent messengers to Cinchon, who was returning to Lima, to sue for peace. They declared themselves willing to submit unconditionally to the Spanish rule. They also offered hostages as guarantees for the honesty of their professions.

Cinchon's heart bled at the thought of the massacre. Although a man who had been in many a battle, he had never seen such bloodshed before. He hid not from himself the fact, that his countrymen had laid themselves open to severe moral censure. A wild beast will slay, but only to satisfy its craving hunger. They murdered simply from bloodthirstiness. Could these unhappy natives ever be won over in this way? Could they ever be converted to Christianity? This was what he most earnestly desired with respect to them, but such experiences as these gave him very little encouragement indeed.

The Indian messengers asked only for the liberation of Huahamac and forgiveness for themselves.

Cinchon would have granted their petition at once but his advisers implored him to first carefully consider the matter. They told him not to forget that Huahamac would plan how to be revenged; that he would not rest until all the Spaniards had been wiped out, or until the Indians themselves were annihilated. They went even further and demanded the chief's execution.

But with this demand they exhausted Cinchon's patience. He grew very angry. In the most earnest and determined manner he refused to accede to their demand, and no one dared again to approach him on this matter. He arrived at Lima very much out of humor, so that even the joyous greeting he received could not cheer him up. Many things however, had happened there during his absence.

Don Cinchon had scarcely left Lima with his troops, when Father Escobar came to the palace. Huahamac was kept a prisoner here in an underground cell, and the priest asked to be permitted to see him, in order to make an effort at his conversion. Donna Dolores, under whose charge the prisoner had been placed by her father, gladly gave the permission, and Escobar spent hours with the chief. But he grew more impatient after each visit. He declared that he had never met with a more stubborn and hardhearted heathen. He began to despair of ever succeeding in his conversion.

This opinion of the priest made a bad impression upon the young lady and especially upon her old "duenna". Nevertheless it did not hinder her from being kind to the prisoner, nor from showing him attentions, and doing everything in her power to ease his lot. She herself bound up his wounds and was overjoyed to see how rapidly they healed. Her coming was indeed a blessing for Huahamac.

He looked upon her as an angel, who had been sent to cheer him, for she was so gentle and kind. She never came to him without showing him some attention, and offering him some relief.

"O, why can I not speak with him," she frequently cried. "I might succeed sooner perhaps, in instilling the principles of our most holy faith, than Father Escobar, against whom he seems to harbor an ill will."

And without a doubt she would have had better success. The prisoner grew more gentle, nay even cheerful, since she began to come to his cell. She never left him without giving expression to her sympathy for him. His wounds rapidly healed under her care, and when Cinchon returned, he found him almost completely recovered.

Huahamac seized his hand as he entered the cell and pressed it against his forehead and then against his breast. He spoke with deep gratefulness of the kindness which had been shown him. Cinchon could not understand his words, and yet he knew what the prisoner wished to say. Upon one occasion when Dolores visited him in company with her father, he pointed up to heaven and then to Dolores. His gesture was too eloquent to be misunderstood. Cinchon looked upon his daughter in happy pride. She was doing what he had asked her to do, and according to the careful training he had given her.

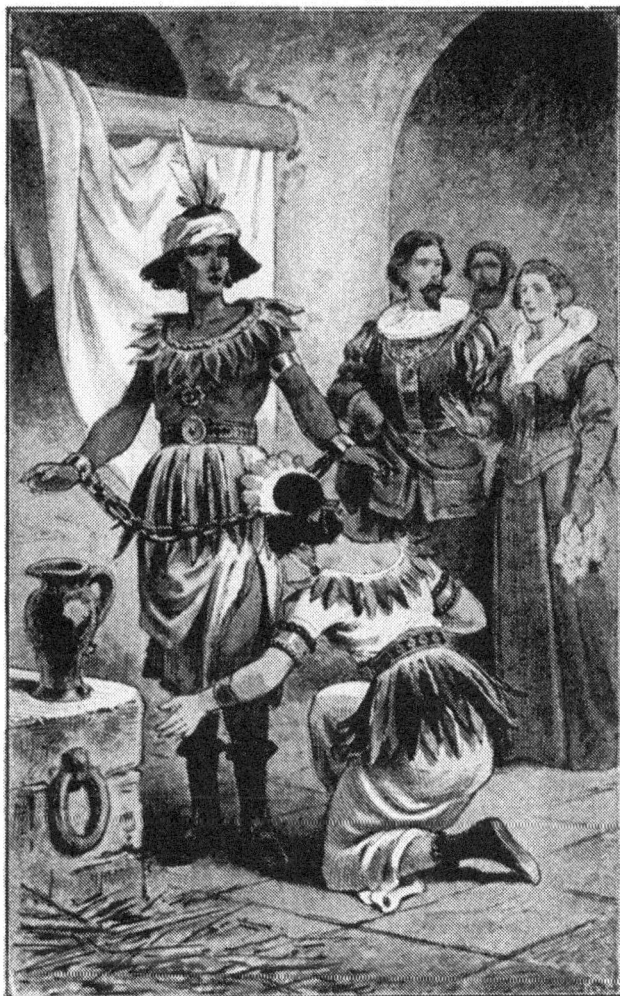

He had declared to the Indian messengers, who had come to him on the homeward march, and with whom he could speak through Perez as interpreter, that he would only then think of making peace with them, if they would again supply Lima with provisions as they had formerly done. On the very day after his return, the great square opposite the palace was crowded with men and women, bringing more supplies than ever before. It was a sign how eager they were to be forgiven and to secure a permanent peace.

Cinchon under such conditions, grew more kindly disposed toward the poor Indians.

However, the more inclined to show mercy the virey grew, the harder his courtiers urged upon him to have Huahamac executed. They told him how absolutely necessary it was for him to make an example.

This moderation, they said, was considered by the Indians to be weakness, nay, they even attributed it to fear. It was Father Escobar alone, who had the courage to urge such opinions before the virey, and he tried every possible means to reach his ends.

The Indians also learned of the virey's inclination to deal mercifully with them. They sent another embassy to him to plead for the liberation of their chief, Huahamac. They emphasized their peaceful sentiments, and as guarantees of their faithfulness, offered to send hostages. Count Cinchon had learned from Escobar, that Huahamac had a daughter, about as old as Dolores, and that the chief clung to her with all his soul, since she was an only child.

Among other hostages he demanded Hualma as hostage for her father. The Indians readily gave their assent.

In a long procession they brought their hostages to

Lima. Then with all the pomp and ceremony customary among the Indians, the treaty of peace was ratified. Huahamac gave his consent to the plan only on the condition, that Hualma should be permitted to remain with Dolores. Cinchon promised him this, and Hualma, herself unbound the fetters of her father.

It was indeed an affecting sight when the young Indian maiden, led by Dolores and accompanied by Cinchon and Perez, entered the cell in which her father was kept.

With a heart-rending cry she fell at his feet. Her lovely eyes streamed with tears. With the greatest difficulty the Indian chief, usually so calm and stolid, kept control of his feelings, which threatened to overpower him.

He drew his child to his bosom and imprinted a kiss upon her forehead. After his fetters had been loosed, he seized Hualma by the hand, and led her over to Dolores. Then he took Dolores' hand and placed it upon Hualma's head. Then he expressed his thanks to Dolores for all the kindness she had shown him, and begged her to treat Hualma like a sister. Most earnestly he spoke to his daughter, and urged her to requite Dolores' kindness to him, by self-sacrificing love and service to her.

After having thus charged his daughter he stepped over to Cinchon. He praised the virey's courage, but above all his merciful spirit. He knew very well, said he, that he had to thank him alone for the fact, that he had not been condemned to die a most cruel death, and would ever remain grateful.

"You are not like the other Spaniards," he continued, "who know no mercy. You are the first one to show the Indians a human heart. Had I known you formerly as I know you now, never would my tomahawk have been raised against your head."

He begged him to treat his beloved child Hualma, tenderly and kindly, and then he departed with the vow, that never again would he take up arms against him.

Perez had faithfully translated these things, and the words of the chief had made an impression even upon him, old Indian fighter though he was. Cinchon took Huahamac's hand, and assured him that he would ever treat Hualma like his own child.

Once more Huahamac embraced his daughter, and then he proudly left the palace in whose prison he had worn the chains of captivity.

The dissatisfaction with the virey's generous treatment of the Indian chief only very gradually, and after a long time disappeared. But he had the satisfaction, that as long as he was at Lima, the peace was not again broken. It is true that the crushing defeat of the Indians in the "Valley of Blood" may have had a great deal to do with this, for their strength had been broken. But long after he had left Peru in order to spend his declining years in the land of his fathers, his name still lingered on the lips of the Indians, as the protector of their people.

CHAPTER III.

In silent, though sad resignation Hualma bore her captivity. She was a captive, even though she moved freely about the palace and enjoyed the companionship of Dolores. The virey's daughter soon came to love her dearly, for Hualma was as gentle as a dove. She seemed to read every wish from Dolores' eyes, and hastened to fulfil it. Yet a keen home-sickness filled her heart. Dolores tried everything to cheer her up, and to make her happy and contented. Unfortunately the chief means for comforting were here lacking. The girls were unable to communicate their thoughts and feelings to each other by speech. Only look and gesture, and the kind and gentle treatment of the Indian maiden, were the means of communication between them.

But Hualma was especially talented. With utmost diligence she tried to learn the Spanish language, and her pains were rewarded. After only six months the two girls were able to make themselves understood to each other. From this time on their intercourse was indeed ideal. They became as closely attached to each other, as if the same mother had given them life. This beautiful relation was due to the fact that both had received from God, their Creator, the same pure, open, generous, mild and tender disposition.

Now Hualma began to grow more cheerful. Her timidity disappeared and she moved more freely in the family circle, a circumstance which made her even more lovable. She still considered herself a servant to Dolores, even though the virey's daughter did her best to dispel such a notion, and tried to lift her to the station she wished her to hold, as companion and friend.

Huahamac had visited her several times. These meetings with her dearly beloved and affectionate father, and the assurance that she might see him often, had overcome her longing for home. Her whole nature seemed to change, and from the sad-eyed mourning Indian maiden, she became sunny and happy.

The fashionable ladies of Lima, who sought so eagerly the society of Dolores, were much displeased at the intimacy which sprang up between the two girls. Even the "duenna" took offence at it, and tried to hinder it in every way. Cinchon however, was delighted with the relation between the two girls, and spoke to the "duenna" so seriously, that she gave up her opposition.

As long as he remained at Lima, Father Escobar tried his best to convert Hualma to Christianity, but the girl felt rather repelled by the stern, harsh man, just as if the repugnance her father had felt against him, had been carried over into her soul. She trembled whenever she saw him.

Cinchon did not venture to interfere with the impetuous man, since such a course might have brought serious consequences with it for the virey, on account of the great influence of the priest. Dolores had been trained to profoundly respect every priest, and she could not bring herself to be unkind, or unfriendly to him.

It was an occasion welcomed by all, when he returned to the mission station of "El Ingenio" in company with another priest of his order. The wealthy people of Lima presented him with rich gifts of money for his work, and he took along with him a number of poor negroes, who were to repair the damage done by the Indians in their late attack.

Now Dolores began a course of instruction which sooner found its way into the Indian girl's heart than the harsh measures of Father Escobar. A stream of holy influence seemed to flow from her soul into the soul of Hualma. Her instruction drove a deeper root, because love prepared the ground into which the seed was sown.

Hualma's eyes were fixed upon the face of her dear friend during these holy and blessed conversations, and not one of the words which the warm, glowing faith of Dolores prompted her to speak was lost.

Hualma soon accompanied her into the lofty cathedral,

where the religious ceremonies made a deep impression upon her. The deepest impressions she received however, when in their own quiet room they would kneel down together, and Dolores would pour forth her sincere words of prayer, just as she was prompted to speak by a devoutly religious heart.

Thus Dolores gently, yet steadily brought the soul of the Indian maiden to the feet of her Saviour; thus she guided her into holy truth, and the road she led her was the more sure, her effort to draw the young soul to Christ the more successful, because a pious, hallowed life went hand in hand with her holy instruction. If the hearts of these young maidens had been bound together in love before, the bond became the firmer now by their common faith in their blessed Redeemer.

The baptism of Hualma was a high festival day for the whole city of Lima. To Dolores it was a higher and more holy festival, for at last she saw realized what she had most earnestly prayed for so long. One might have expected that Huahamac would have grown furious when he learned that his daughter had accepted the faith of the Spaniards. This was not the case however, for the kind treatment he had received at the hands of Cinchon, as he often said, had changed his heart. From a bitter enemy he had been changed into a devoted friend, since he had experienced Don Cinchon's generosity. He came to Lima very often. He learned more and more to love and honor Dolores and her father, for he saw how they treated his daughter not as an hostage, but as a friend and sister, as a child of the family. In this house he beheld the rich fruits of a sincere Christian faith, and he no longer was opposed to what Hualma told him of her intention, for his heart was reconciled to a faith that could lead to such noble deeds.

Huahamac was a very sensible person. His heart had so much good in it, that he formed an exception among his people. He was constantly exerting his influence for good, for the uplifting of the Indians. Whenever he came Cinchon received him most cordially. The shrewd, keen-eyed Indian saw that this friendliness was not a mask, which the virey merely wore in order to hide his true feelings; that it was not an artificial kindness, practiced merely in order to win him, the powerful Inca, for the purposes of the Spaniards. That would have repelled him. But his heart was won by the frank, and honest, and heartfelt kindness which was uniformly shown him, and he blessed the day which brought him into a closer contact with the virey, and led his child into Cinchon's house, while his people and their priests cursed the Spaniards and the defeat which they had suffered through them. If Huahamac had not been an Inca, a descendant of the ancient family of the rulers of Peru, whom the natives revered almost as a God, he would have lost all his influence as chief. Again and again he urged the maintenance of peace. He pointed out to his people that the Spaniards held an over-whelming majority, and that every attempt to overcome them by war, must lead to inevitable defeat.

"Children of the Sun" was what the Peruvians called their Incas. They were accustomed to show blind obedience to their will. If they gave in to Huahamac however, it was because they felt themselves too weak to take up arms after the crushing defeat they had sustained. But they submitted with the impotent rage of the defeated and oppressed.

Huahamac's relations with Don Cinchon were product-ive of much good in another direction also. It was he who reported to the virey every act of brutality which a Spaniard had perpetrated upon the natives. The hatred and fury of the defeated people could easily be fanned into fresh flames by these things. But whenever he made such a communication, the virey at once took steps to mete out justice, and the offender was made to feel the sharpness of the laws. Huahamac never failed to bring such acts of justice to the notice of his people in order to create confidence in the noble virey. He called him the "Father of the Indians". While his efforts were not successful with all, yet he won over so many that it seemed as if peace would be secured for a long time for blood-washed Peru. This hope was a source of great happiness for Don Cinchon. His rule was a period of blessing a circumstance which was recognized in Lima, as the Indians also had come to know it.

The happiness of the noble virey seemed perfect. The foundations of his happiness were peace without, developing trade with the Indians, favor in Madrid, and the joy, which as a father, he took in his child, Dolores.

Yet — — — when is man's happiness unclouded? When are the heavens perfectly clear? When is man's joy absolutely complete?

CHAPTER IV.

Since the conquest of Peru by Pizarro it had been a most deplorable fact, that more Spaniards perished in consequence of the unhealthy climate, than by the arrows of the Indians. All along the coast of Peru they died of malaria fever, after a prolonged illness. No medical skill, nor the most carefully regulated life, could protect

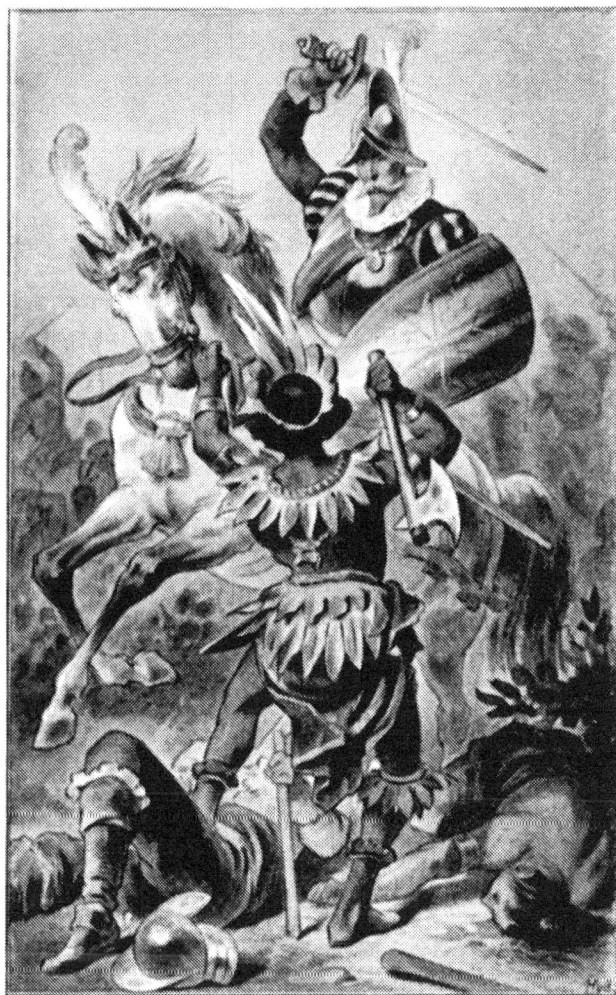

the European against this fever, which only the strongest constitutions seemed able to withstand, and even these sometimes succumbed to it. Those who were attacked by it, dragged themselves along, their faces haggard, their limbs trembling, their complexion a yellowish brown, and all of them sooner or later, became victims of the horrible disease from which there seemed no escape. Even when a patient dragged himself aboard a vessel to seek a more favorable climate, he did not always succeed in shaking it off. He bore the germs of the malady with him from the first chill, and like a messenger of death was that first cold chill which shook his body. The Indians noted this wasting away of their oppressors with a mocking smile. For a long time the Spaniards were bound to dwell in the fever districts along the coast, because they did not succeed in founding secure towns farther up in the highlands and mountains. Besides the Indians gave them little opportunity for rest, or even for the care of the sick, and so it seemed as if in this way they would be relieved of their haughty oppressors, and that the grave would swallow up the last Spaniard.

This was the bold, but unjustified hope of a people who had been made wretched by the Spaniards. The greed for gold characteristic of the Spaniards of that time, brought new numbers of oppressors to the shores of Peru. Neither the murderous battles with the Peruvians, nor the destructive malaria fever could prevent the steady stream of fortune hunters from pouring into Peru. They believed it to be the land where all their hopes would be realized. They called it El Dorado, under which name they pictured to themselves a city, nay even a country, where everything which a man needed in his house, was made of pure gold. Such fabulous tales as these had inflamed the brains of those old Spaniards in a most incredible manner, and filled them with a longing to find this El Dorado. Whoever could get away tried to reach distant Peru. The dangers and difficulties of the long journey were not considered, and the greed for gold overcame even the fear of almost certain death by the malaria fever of the coast.

Everyone thought: "I will escape the dangers; I will not get the fever; I will find El Dorado." This was the sorcery by which the goldhunters were lured to the deadly place.

It was wonderful that the Indians rarely contracted the fever, or if one did catch it, he recovered in a remarkably short time.

Were they immune as natives of the place? Could they easier overcome it? Or did they perhaps possess a medicine which secured them against it, or healed them when attacked?

The Spaniards were most anxious to get clearness on these points. After Lima had been built, and regular intercourse with the Indians had been established, they had ample opportunity afforded them to make observations. They were all of the opinion, and this was confirmed by experience, that the Indians were just as frequently attacked by the malady as the Spaniards, as soon as they came into the northern fever-zone of the coast. They grew weak just as rapidly, but just as soon as they could come together with their Indian friends, or just as soon as they could get into the woods of the mountains, the germs of the disease were destroyed, and they recovered after a longer or shorter period, according to the length of time they had suffered from the disease. Every means were tried to discover the secret. Once in a while intimate friendships sprang up between Spaniards and Peruvians, but the secret was not found out. Even the most cruel torture failed to draw it out. Yet, without a doubt, there was such a secret. It was most probable that terrible oaths, and the fearful threats of the Indian priests closed the mouths of the people. It was possible also that the priests, who among the Indians were the physicians as well, alone knew the secret. Who could get positive answers to such questions?

Thus every attempt to find out the secret failed. The Indians who possessed it enjoyed its decided advantages, while without it the Spaniards wasted away and died.

Experience had taught the Europeans that the climate was healthier and safer at a certain altitude above the coast. This had determined the selection of the site upon which the city of Lima had been built, which lay quite far up the mountain. They had hoped thus to escape the dreadful fever of the swamps. But the experiences of the future were a disappointment of their hopes. Two things endangered life in Lima, the climate and the frequent earthquakes.

The climate of Lima was agreeable in a way, but it was not at all healthy. From April to October a heavy mist settled over the city and the surrounding country. The skies always began to be obscured in April. The morning hours were dreary and disagreeably cool. The rays of the noontide sun at this time still succeeded in penetrating through the veil of mists, but by the middle of this month they had already grown so dense, as to completely hide the sun's face. The mist was ever the cause of an intense humidity, although the temperature was not lowered in the least. The mist lingered along until October, then its density grew gradually less, until at last it disappeared altogether.

This was the dangerous season of the year. Besides being menaced by other contagious diseases, malaria seized upon the inhabitants, claiming many victims.

It was a peculiar thing that Europeans rarely took the fever upon first coming to Lima. Only after they had lived there for a while, and already began to comfort themselves with the thought, that they had accustomed themselves to the manner of living required by the local conditions, and that they had grown used to the climate, only then were they taken with it. Very often the terrible tribute required by the treacherous climate was not demanded before the second year of residence, and generally was paid by death.

The inhabitants of Lima had therefore, been bitterly disappointed in their hopes. But a more grievous disappointment still was in store for them. The terrible and frequent earthquakes were also believed to be overcome by the high location of the city, but the future showed Lima to be in the very centre of the zone of these disturbances. It was seldom that any length of time passed without the town being visited by an earthquake. These usually proved quite destructive, and always filled the inhabitants with terror. In the course of time Lima had to pass through terrible visitations by earthquakes. There were times during which not a day, not a night passed without a more or less violent shock.

Cinchon had now been viceroy of Peru for several years, and had not yet been attacked by the deadly malaria fever. In fact, his health had not been affected so frequently here in this new country, as had been the case during his residence in Spain. And so he began to think himself immune. He believed that the strength of his constitution made him secure against any attack. He was very much concerned about Dolores however, who was a frail and delicate creature. He warned her repeatedly to be very careful so as not to contract colds, and to avoid eating the juicy and cooling fruits of the native trees. He watched over her himself with all the care of an affectionate father, and if the slightest indisposition showed itself, at once summoned the best physicians of Lima.

But all this care could not prevent, that the rosy cheeks of the young girl gradually grew paler and paler, a circumstance which filled her father with secret terror. He consulted with the leading physicians, and their recommendations were followed out most conscientiously. In the meantime Dolores appeared to be well and was in the best of spirits, and so her father began to hope that she would escape the fever, and by this hope permitted himself to be lulled into a feeling of security.

When April for the second time since her arrival, began to spread its misty mantle over the city, Dolores began to feel an increasing weariness. Her sleep was no more so refreshing as it used to be. It happened that occasionally, even on very warm days, she experienced a slight chill, but it was so slight and of such brief duration, that it was more like a shiver. These forerunners of the terrible fever would not escape the eye of an experienced observer, especially since her appetite also began to fail. There were two persons who observed these ill-boding signs, Cinchon and Hualma, who were attached to Dolores with a love, capable of any sacrifice. Filled with grave presentiments, she tried in every way to cheer her up. With the increasing weakness of her body, however, Dolores also began to sink into a melancholy frame of mind. Hualma could no longer cheer her. Even her Indian dances and native songs which had formerly given Dolores so much pleasure, now failed to arouse her from her languor. Frequently when the young Peruvian knew herself to be alone and unobserved, she would wring her hands in agony of spirit, while the tears streamed from her large, lustrous black eyes. Then she would sink into brooding, and would give expression to the grief of her soul in loud sighs. When she recovered her composure she carefully removed all traces of her sorrow before returning to Dolores, who spent the greater part of the day reclining on a couch.

Cinchon also tried just as hard to hide his anxiety from his daughter, who often gazed at him with a most peculiar sorrowful, questioning glance. The physicians exhausted their doubtful art. Soon the unmistakable symptoms of the destroying fever were apparent to all.

Cinchon would not move from her bedside after that. Out of the wreck of his life's happiness, Dolores was all that was left to him. And now he had to see her wasting away without hope of recovery. He knew the disease well enough to be convinced that Dolores must inevitably succumb to it. For this malady the physicians had not yet found a cure, and the medicines they employed against it, were without any effect whatever.

Thus the deepest sorrow and heaviest care had entered the palace of the virey, where a happiness had reigned since the coming of Dolores, such as it had not seen before. Greater sorrow, greater care than this, man can not know on earth. The whole palace seemed as if died out. The servants noiselessly moved about. No one dared to speak a loud word, for fear of disturbing her, whom they all held dear in love and reverence.

The visits of those kind citizens, who came to show their sympathy with the noble young lady in her suffering, could not be received, however well they were meant. Rest and absolute quiet were the most necessary things required for the patient.

The business of state was transacted by the virey in the lower appartment of his palace, so that no sound whatever might disturb the sufferer. So great was the sympathy with the sufferings of the young lady in Lima, that the Plaza Major, the great square between the virey's palace and the cathedral, was voluntarily deserted. The market which it was customary to hold there, was transferred to another, distant square; and instead of taking their evening promenade there as they were used to do, the people went along the Alameda, beyond the Gate of Callao. In every way they thus also showed the tenderest consideration for the father in his sorrow, for they all held him in highest esteem. Unfortunately the efforts of the physicians were as fruitless, as all this considerate love of the people. The disease steadily progressed, and vitality was being exhausted. The time could not be far distant any more, when the young life would have to succumb to the treacherous malady.

It is a sad experience of life, that our troubles never come singly.

Cinchon also was to learn that his anxiety for his child was not to be his only trouble. He had never been quite relieved of the unrest which had been caused by the excitement due to the outbreak of the Indians. Now that his daughter was taken so critically ill, this disquiet, or rather nervousness began to increase. Even at the time of the Indian outbreak he had suffered from loss of sleep. Disquieting thoughts drove it from him. When Dolores began to suffer from the fever, he gave himself no rest at all. To all the multitude of cares connected with his position, came this great anxiety for his child. Was it to be wondered at, that all this began to seriously effect his health?

He felt the approach of the sickness, but the iron will of the man held back its outbreak. But when the time of the heavy fogs arrived, the disease broke out in a much more dangerous and irresistible form.

He made a desperate attempt to hide the truth from Dolores, but of course, did not long succeed in doing so. He had been attacked much more severely than she, and sooner than she was compelled to take to his bed.

Hualma now became the tireless, devoted nurse of both sufferers. The clearer she recognized the progress of the disease, the more anxious she became. A fatal ending seemed absolutely certain, since none of the medicines employed by the physicians of Lima took any effect whatever.

It was just at this critical time, that Huahamac, impelled by the longing to see his child, came to Lima.

Hualma saw him coming and ran to meet him.

"You look ill! You are weeping, my dear child," said he. "What has happened? Speak!"

"O, my father," cried the heart-broken girl, "Dolores, my dearly beloved Dolores, is lying hopelessly ill with the fever. Her life is like to a light burning out. Soon she will surrender her pure soul into the hands of her God. But this is not all! The virey also, who loves me like a father, the blessed benefactor of Peru, he who saved your life, he also has been taken with this terrible disease, which mercilessly slays these strangers. If Dolores should die, my heart shall break; for I do not care to live without her. If the virey should die, he will be followed by a Spaniard without a heart, without mercy, and our poor people will again become the victims of pitiless and cruel persecution, as was the case formerly, according to what you have told me. Dear father, must they then die?"

These words were accompanied by a look from the beautiful eyes of the girl, so beseeching, so sorrowful, that it entered into the very soul of the chief. Still Huahamac remained silent for a long time.

"Father, will you not answer your child?" cried the girl in great excitement.

"You know, Hualma, what an oath binds my tongue," he answered slowly in a most sorrowful tone.

"An oath made to destroy, to kill the noblest men, is a most guilty thing before God," she cried.

Huahamac again remained silent, but his face became clouded as by heavy trouble.

"Let us go to them," he said, seizing her hand. Together they entered Don Cinchons apartment.

Huahamac drew back in fright, as he beheld the wasted frame of the once powerful man. Cinchon was scarcely able to give his hand to the chief, so feeble had he grown during the brief time of his illness. His face had grown thin; his eyes lay deep in their sockets, and his skin was frightfully yellow.

Huahamac was deeply moved at the sight.

"I am afraid that the end has come for my dear Dolores and for me," said the virey. "There is no cure for this wasting fever. Our physicians have tried everything, but nothing takes effect, nothing helps. Alas! why did I ever summon her to Peru?"

The tone of his voice showed the intense sorrow which filled the soul of the virey. Hualma took his hands between hers and leaned her head against the wall. The tears streamed from her eyes. Huahamac looked upon him in sincere sympathy.

"We are not quite as far as that," he said firmly. He had learned to speak a little Spanish.

"You foolish man," said the virey, "do you also wish to deceive me as the doctors are trying to do? Do you think that I am not aware, that no man ever recovered, who had the fever as severe as I have it? Do you really think that the delicate constitution of my child, can resist this treacherous malady? No, Huahamac, I do not give myself over to false hopes, which must be disappointed. Nay, I consider it wrong to do so. I must think of my end, and prepare for it, in order that I may stand before the eternal Judge of my days. There is one comfort for me, namely that my beloved Dolores will soon be with me in the eternal kingdom of my God."

Huahamac was deeply moved by the words he heard.

The physician entered at this moment and found Don Cinchon somewhat excited, and weaker in consequence.

"You have spoken with the Indian too long," he said. "This is very harmful to you."

Hualma understood the words of the physician. She gently drew her father from the room. Once outside the door he released his hand.

"I do not wish to see Dolores," he said. "It might do her harm."

Then Hualma threw herself upon her knees before him. She lifted up her hands to him beseechingly and whispered:

"O my father, have mercy upon her and upon your own child!"

"Hualma," he cried, "you do not know what you are asking. By the sun I have sworn never to reveal the cure to a Spaniard."

"It is a godless oath, which in itself is a sin before God," cried the girl springing to her feet. "You have sworn it by the creature instead of by Him, who gave it existence and life. In your blindness, father, you swore it to the destruction of your fellowmen. It is your solemn duty to break that oath, unless you would load heavier guilt still upon your soul."

"Did they not torture us mercilessly? Did they not murder our wives and children, and our best warriors relentlessly? Have they not robbed us of the land of our fathers?" he asked with quivering voice.

"It is their fault," returned the girl with earnestness, "but Jesus Christ, the Son of the living God, our Saviour, says: 'Bless them that curse you, do good to them that hate you, and pray for them which despitefully use, and persecute you; that ye may be the children of your Father which is in heaven: for he maketh his sun to rise on the evil and on the good, and sendeth rain on the just and on the unjust!'"

"Does He say that?" the Indian asked with a peculiar tone of astonishment.

"Yes, my father, these are His words. But more than that, this is what He did during His life on earth. He did this while His enemies were crucifying Him under unspeakable tortures. He prayed for His enemies: 'Father forgive them, they know not what they do!'"

The Indian's head fell upon his breast. He stood thus for a while as if he were a statue carved out of stone, deeply engaged in thought. Suddenly he tore himself away from Hualma, and hastily left the palace. Hualma wished to hurry after him, but he ran like some wild animal pursued by the hunter. She could not catch up with him, and by the time she emerged from the palace, he had disappeared in one of the streets leading into the Plaza Major.

She hurried back into the palace and up to her apartment, closing the door behind her. Here she threw herself upon her knees, and folding her hands, she lifted eye and hand to heaven in her appeal. Her lips moved slightly, but no sound was heard; only this much the ear might have distinguished: "Lord, Lord, enlighten him by Thy Spirit, and move his soul to a blessed determination."

When she again became composed, and had removed

the tear-stains from her face, she left her apartment, in order to prepare a cool, refreshing drink for the patients, from the juice of some delicious fruit, which is found in such abundance on the mountain-sides of Peru. She alone knew how to prepare this drink, and from her hands alone Dolores and her father would receive it. Now again she brought it to the patients in golden cups, and affectionate looks and grateful words were an ample reward for the true and faithful girl.

CHAPTER V.

The Indians of Peru had long been acquainted with a positive remedy for malaria fever. This was the bark of a certain tree, known to us as Peruvian bark. They had used the cure in the treatment of every case occurring among them since time immemorial, and since the treatment became known in Europe, physicians recognize in it the only reliable means with which to fight this treacherous fever. I will have to speak of this tree to my readers, because the thread of the story compels me. Let me first relate to you what the Indians of Peru tell about the discovery of the healing properties of the bark of this tree.

A certain Peruvian had been guilty of a crime, which was punishable by death, according to the laws of his people, and the Inca, or ruler of the people, had spoken the irrevocable sentence. The Peruvian however, belonged to a distinguished and powerful family, who could not endure the thought that one of their number should be executed as a criminal, and thus a great disgrace be brought upon them all. They put forth every effort to aid him to escape, and they succeeded. Pachicamak was the name of the criminal. He fled into the almost impassable fastnesses of the mighty mountain range, which runs through the country. The Inca of Peru exhausted every means in vain in his effort to again get him into his power. His hiding-place could not be discovered for the simple reason that it was not a single place, for the fugitive was sly enough not to remain in hiding too long in one place. The regions that he sought out were the wildest and most unknown parts of the Andes mountains, or the Cordillera de los Andes, as the Spaniards called the range. There he hid himself in deep gorges, in caves, or in impenetrable thickets. He never suffered from lack of food because the favored land produces an abundance of wholesome fruit, which everywhere grows wild. His arrow never failed to hit when he shot, and to bring down the lama, which lives in that climate, and whose flesh is very nourishing and strengthening.

But this restless life in the damp gorges of the mountains, finally began to have an evil effect upon his health. In consequence of the dampness, of sleeping in the open air, of drinking different kinds of water, and of often eating the cool, refreshing fruits of trees, he was seized with the fever common in those parts. He quickly understood that the end of his days was quite near. With the progress of the disease it grew harder for him to travel. He sought out a spot therefore, where he erected a hut of moss, and now comfortless and forsaken, he determined to await his end. Whenever the sun shone near his hut, he dragged himself forth to enjoy some of its warmth, without exposing himself to its burning rays.

A rocky wall, thickly overgrown with shrubbery, afforded him an excellent opportunity for this. From this point he could look into a little valley running off to one side. He noticed there a peculiar kind of tree, which he had not seen elsewhere in the Andes mountains, although his eye saw the familiar plants and trees of his home on every side.

These trees, growing together in groups near the edge of the dense forests of trees of different species, attained a height of between thirty and forty feet. Their trunks were covered with a bark which was sometimes of a greenish, then again of a brownish, or redish-brown color, and very rough. The branches grew straight out from the trunk, and had beautiful leaves, of a shining green, at all seasons of the year. At the ends of the branches there grew bunches of bell-shaped flowers, upon which the eye rested with as much pleasure, as the nostrils found in inhaling their lovely scent.

Pachicamak easily distinguished different species. Although the general shape of the trees, the bark and the leaves was almost the same with all, the bunches of flowers differed, sometimes being pure white, then again of a bright red color.

The fruit formed a capsule, but uneatable, of a bitter, disagreeable taste. At the time Pachicamak lay sick and weak in the mountains, these fine trees were in full bloom, and their sweet scent as well as their beauty, as they hung under the protecting roof of the shining fresh leaves, refreshed, and strengthened him.

As he lay there thinking of the nearness of his end, he could not entirely repress his longing for father, mother, brothers and sisters. He felt the need of at least seeing a living being. It was seldom however, at that height, that he saw a bird or any animal; only the giant-bird of the Andes, the condor, he occasionally beheld, hovering in almost immeasurable heights, whence it searched out its prey, upon which it pounced like a dart of lightning. Thus time dragged on heavily for him, and had there not dwelt in his youthful soul that love for life characteristic of those of his age, he would have longed for death to come sooner, than his disease seemed to threaten. Just this slow progress of his disease, with the certainly of its outcome, made the future appear more and more dreary to him. One day he again lay propped up against the rocky wall, following his gloomy thoughts, when he saw a lama creeping along, quite without fear, for it did not see him. It was very lean and its gait was tottering. Its breath was short, and its flanks rose and fell quickly. The animal was evidently suffering from a disease similar to that of Pachicamak. He observed it closely, and to his astonishment saw it eat the bark of the tree, whose beauty he had so often admired.

For quite a number of days the animal appeared every morning and ate of the bark of the tree. From day to day the healing effect of the remedy became more apparent. The appearance of the animal improved, it became sportive, and its strength increased, until finally it no longer came.

"How?" cried Pachicamak. "Should not the bark perhaps help me as well? I must die a slow death from exhaustion at all events. I shall try it."

He tried to drag himself near to one of the trees. With great difficulty he broke off some of the bark and began to chew it. It required the utmost selfcontrol for the taste was exceedingly bitter, and it drew together his mouth by its sharpness.

When he had repeated this for several days he thought to his great delight, that he noticed an improvement in his condition. He then steadily continued the use of the strangely discovered remedy, and had the satisfaction of seeing his malady entirely disappear.

When he had completely recovered, he gathered a great quantity of the healing bark, and then approached the place where his tribe was dwelling.

One day he met a friend in the forest, who told him that the Inca, who had condemned him to death, had been seized with the fever and was near his end. It flashed through Pachicamak's mind that he might make his remedy the ground of his salvation. He asked his friend to tell the Inca, that he was in the possession of an infallible remedy for the fever. He would heal him on the condition that pardon would be granted, and if he failed, he would come and voluntarily lay his head upon the executioner's block.

His friend did what Pachicamak bade him to do. The message aroused in the soul of the Inca, a strong love of life. He vowed solemnly that Pachicamak should be a free man, if his cure succeeded. And so he was summoned to the court of the Inca.

But the bark had become quite dry and hard by this time, and he tried to find a way to make it easy to take. The idea came to him to grind it to powder. This he did. The Inca faithfully took the powder and in a short time had completely recovered, and so had many others who had suffered from the fever, and to whom the remedy had been administered. Thus a cure had been discovered, and for centuries the remedy proved sure against the fevers, which the Indians no longer dreaded.

When the Spaniards under Pizarro conquered Peru, the fever showed itself as the most reliable ally of the Indians. They saw the Spaniards dying helplessly, and they bound themselves by an oath, whose breaking meant an awful death, never to reveal the remedy to a Spaniard. And this oath they kept faithfully. The Jesuits tried in vain to coax the secret from those whom they converted;

in vain the viceroys subjected Indians to the most terrible torture in order to draw it from them, they would die under their sufferings, but the seal could not be removed from their lips. They kept their oath.

Hualma also knew the legend of Pachicamak. She had frequently seen the almost miraculous effect of the remedy. She knew that it consisted of the powdered bark of a tree growing in a distant part of the Cordillera de los Andes, but the tree she did not know, nor the place where it grew. She would have shunned no difficulties, no dangers in order to obtain the healing bark for those persons, whom she loved so dearly. However, she had most earnestly pleaded with her. father, and she had noted what a deep impression her words had made upon him. Upon this fact, but especially upon the evident change in his way of thinking which she had observed, she based her hopes, that he would bring the remedy by which the virey and her beloved Dolores would be saved. The change in her father's views was also the source of a blessed happiness for her. The frequent visits he made in the palace of the virey were in themselves a proof of this change. But she learned it more from the high regard and kindly affection with which he used to speak of the virey and Dolores. From occasional remarks which he made, she also learned, that he was a frequent visitor at the Jesuit settlements, the so-called missions, which had been established for the purpose of carrying on the work of converting the Indians. He spoke in terms of highest admiration of those men, who had given up the more comfortable life of the cities, in order to settle in the lonely mountains, for the purpose of carrying on the work of evangelizing the Indians. He knew that this was connected with infinite hardships, and required great devotion, many sacrifices and much self-denial; and sometimes they had to endure even sufferings

4

and persecutions. She had with great joy observed, that he had come more often of late, and had frequently asked her about the teachings of the Saviour. She could not but see how earnestly he had listened to her, when she explained to him the moral wrong of the Indian's pledge to keep from the Spaniards the knowledge of the cure for the fever. And finally she had noted the deep impression made upon him by the words of the Saviour: "Bless them which curse you; do good to them which hate you and persecute you." She well knew his earnest manner in which he would often ponder over a matter for a long time, if it interested him. All these things supported her in that hope in which she daily prayed to her God and Saviour, and in the confidence that her prayers would be heard.

However, a week rolled by and he did not return. The disease of Cinchon and Dolores made slow but steady progress, and still there came no help. Her anxiety increased day by day. Often she would wring her hands as if in despair, and her prayers were a wrestling of the soul with her Lord.

A hundred times she resolved to go to her father, and a hundred times she had to give up her purpose. She was a hostage for her people, and well she knew the dreadful consequences of such a step, which would be looked upon as flight, as breaking her pledge. And who would nurse the sick while she was away? The "duenna" of her friend Dolores was an old woman, unable even with the best of will, to nurse both patients, and she felt that she could not entrust so sacred and responsible an office to the negro slaves. They were slaves and lacked the self sacrificing love, which alone made one competent for such a service.

Ah. Hualma had no idea of the battles Huahamac

had to fight. He had been brought up in the religion and customs of his fathers, and never once had the thought entered his mind that it was wrong to take that oath, which was part of the usages of his people, and which was rooted in their hatred of the Spaniards, their merciless oppressors.

He had already departed from the ways of his people when he began going to the missions to listen to the words of the preachers. According to the views of his people he was already faithless because he loved and honored a Spaniard. And yet — — — could he refuse to follow his conscience and his clear understanding? He had himself known two noble Spaniards, the excellent Las Casas, whom his father already had honored, and the virey together with his pure, angelic daughter Dolores. This had struck root in his heart, and he began to search for other good points with the missionaries, which would be in favor of the Spaniards. But he was compelled to bury such opinions deep in his own heart, and he did it most successfully. To these things came his conversations with Hualma, which introduced a kindling fire into his soul. He sought solitude in order to ponder over many questions and to gain clearness, to come to some conclusion. He was entirely occupied with these things, until at last the highest Spirit broke all fetters, and out of his severe conflicts, he emerged a victor.

Now he set out for the place where those remarkable trees grew. The way was long, and the dangers for him were great, since none of his own tribe must have any suspicion of his intentions. Already the priests were watching him. They were wroth with him, because he so often went to Lima to the palace of the virey; they all knew about the illness of the virey and his daughter.

He had an excellent excuse for going to the palace.

His only daughter was there and his heart urged him to seek her, to be where she was. But because he knew himself watched, it was a good thing that for so long a time he had not been at Lima. He would have to try to get the feverbark, as the Indians called their remedy, into Hualma's hands as cautiously as possible, and then avoid Lima and any intercourse of the virey's palace for a long time.

There came a dark night during the foggy season. Hualma in her anxiety had retired to her room for a few minutes, while the "duenna" watched in the sick-room. She leaned her weary head against the windowpane, and the grief of her soul found vent in her sighs and tears.

Suddenly she heard the door of her room open almost noiselessly. Quickly turning about she inquired: "Who is it?"

"I," answered Huahamac in the Peruvian language. She at once recognized the sound of her father's voice, and hastened to him to throw her arms around his neck.

"Have you come at last?" she cried. "Do you at last bring me help?"

"I have brought it," Huahamac answered softly, as he placed a small package in her hand. Then he gently loosed her arms and said: "My time is short, let us speak of the most necessary things. You know well the conditions. You are aware that if it becomes known that I have given you the remedy my life is forfeited. No one, not even the patients, nor the "duenna", must know from whom you have received the bark. The "duenna" must not even know that you are administering it, for old women are talkative. Make the virey and Dolores solemnly promise to be absolutely silent about the matter. The doctors also must not be permitted to suspect its use. Let them think that their miserable remedies have saved the patients.

Never forget for a moment that your father's life is at stake."

He then gave her specific instructions about the proper use of the remedy. Once more he embraced her and kissed her on the forehead.

"Do not worry," said he, "if you should not see me for the next six months. Precaution forbids my coming to you for a long time."

With these words he glided through the door like a shadow and was gone. The overjoyed girl fell upon her knees and gave thanks to the Lord, who had made all things well. She commended her father to the care of the all-merciful God, and prayed for His blessing upon the remedy. Then she hurried away to the patients.

It was an easy matter to persuade the "duenna" to leave the sick-room. The old woman had been up with the patients the previous night, in order to give the girl a chance to get some rest after the many nights she had spent in watching. And so Hualma urged her to go and get a little sleep.

After the "duenna" had gone, Hualma told the virey and his daughter everything her father had said.

A new courage entered into the hearts of these two who had believed themselves hopelessly ill. They cheerfully promised to keep the secret inviolate. Both at once took a dose of the remedy with an eagerness, which in itself seemed to offer a guarantee for a good result.

The two physicians who had been treating the patients, came once more late that evening. They were amazed at the change in the condition of their charges. They had last seen them utterly hopeless, they found them full of hope. They had been deeply despondent, and were now cheerful to a degree which they had not expected.

They, of course, ascribed this to the medicines they

had employed. They left with the urgent injunction to most carefully continue their use. They extended the comfort, that although the physical condition of their patients did not seem to be much improved, yet their spirits had revived, which was an excellent sign, and the sure proof that they had found the proper remedy at last.

It was necessary to leave them under this illusion. Hualma now began to pour away the medicines in the measure in which she ought to have administered them. Naturally however, she gave the patients nothing by way of treatment, except the remedy of her father, and strictly in accordance with the directions he had given her.

The continued use of the dry, powdered Peruvian bark soon showed itself effective. Aided by their renewed courage, the spirits of the patients wonderfully revived. The fevers daily grew less severe in their attacks, and strength returned visibly. With these favorable symptoms cheerfulness and confidence increased, and the improvement was so steady as to leave no doubt of a speedy recovery.

The two physicians were jubilant over the success of their treatment, and loudly boasted of it throughout Lima. The constant intercourse between the Indians and the citizens of the capitol, made it impossible to confine this astounding news to Lima. The Indians wondered greatly, but no one for an instant suspected Huahamac, who had not been in the city since long before the recovery of the virey and his daughter. When he heard the news his heart rejoiced, and he gave thanks to the God his daughter worshipped, and Whom he was also trying to find.

CHAPTER VI.

The virey and his daughter were very highly respected and much beloved by the citizens of Lima and in fact of all the Spanish settlements in Peru, when they therefore, as soon as they were permitted to go out again, took their way to the cathedral to thank God for their recovery, the occasion was made a festival of rejoicing by great throngs.

The Plaza Major was crowded with men and women and children of all classes on that Sunday morning. After the long period of fog, the sun also for the first time again broke through. Everyone was anxious to see the two, who had been healed in so wonderful a manner, and to give them a proof of the general rejoicing at their recovery.

The virey stepped from the great door of the palace; Dolores walked at his right, and Hualma at his left. The two convalescents appeared healthy, even though they still showed traces of the serious and protracted illness through which they had passed. All eyes were turned toward them as they issued from the palace, and a great shout from the people greeted them, while the sound of the mighty cathedral bells mingled with the joyous greetings of the people. Cinchon waved his thanks, bowing in every direction, and the expression of his face showed how much he was pleased with this demonstration of the kindly feeling of the populace for him. The three had now reached the Plaza, where the people formed a passage-way for them. A great number of young girls of the best families of the city came forward, carrying neat baskets filled with flowers, which they strewed over the way. Thus they crossed the square. At the entrance of the cathedral they were received by the archbishop of Lima and many priests. After they had taken their places in the choir, and the people had streamed in, filling every bit of space in the great sanctuary, the solemn services began. After the religious ceremonies were over, the three were escorted back to the palace under the same ovations with which they had been received. At the palace the city officials had assembled themselves and formally extended their congratulations to the virey. Far into the night the visits continued of those who desired to extend personal congratulations, while upon the square the people made holiday, giving expression to their joy by singing and dancing.

It was late when the virey at last entered his apartments accompanied by two negroes bearing candles. His first glance fell upon an Indian standing in the silent, dignified attitude characteristic of his race. Cinchon at once recognized Huahamac. He quickly dismissed the negroes, then hastened toward the Indian, and threw his arms about him in a long embrace, for in the fulness of his heart, he found it impossible to utter a word.

Huahamac was deeply affected by this proof of sincere gratefulness, such as no Indian ever before had received from the haughty Spaniards.

Only after he had recovered his selfcontrol, was Cinchon able to give expression to the feelings, which filled his heart, and out of whose fulness his mouth now ran over.

"Ah, I know how to appreciate what you have done for me," he cried, "and never, never shall I forget it."

"Do not thank me," replied the Indian deeply moved, "but let my people reap the fruit of your kindness. Continue to treat them kindly, and they will bless your name, and it shall be deeply engraven upon their hearts."

Cinchon promised this with a solemn and sacred vow.

"But you," he said, "you are the saviour of my child and myself!"

Again he threw his arms about the Indian, warmly embracing him. Then he summoned Dolores and Hualma. The latter had been anxiously looking about for her father, without having been able to discover him. Now she found him just as Dolores, having seized his hand, covered it with tears of gratefulness. At a glance she saw how deeply he was affected, and she too threw her arms about him in affectionate embrace.

These scenes moved Cinchon more deeply than all the congratulations which he had received. The four sat together until after midnight, when Huahamac tore himself away, in order to return to his home among the mountains.

It was a grand, happy day which Cinchon had passed, and his soul was filled with holy impulses. He again vowed before his God to solemnly keep the promises he had given Huahamac, and he did keep them even under the most trying conditions.

He very frequently communicated with Huahamac, although the chief came to him only secretly, and ever departed under cover of the night.

He learned from him many things about which he had before vainly sought to fully inform himself. Huahamac was thoroughly acquainted with the condition of his people, especially in their relations with the Spaniards. The virey became acquainted through the chief with many deep-rooted abuses, and he saw how cruelly the Indians had been treated. He saw how the causes of bloody wars were to be sought on the side of the Spaniards alone. This information led him to devise new legal measures for the protection of the Indians and for the prevention of violence, which the Spaniards were constantly committing against the natives, because heretofore the guilty ones had never been punished, but the blame had always been put upon the Indians. This had led more than one of his predecessors to commit acts of cruelty, even though otherwise gentle in their rule. But these acts only deepened the hatred against the Spaniards, and after awhile another one of those bloody conflicts would break out, such as he had himself experienced, whereby the misery of the Indians however, was merely increased.

But these laws and regulations for the protection of the Indians, which filled them with gratefulness, had the opposite effect upon the Spaniards. The more the Indians honored and revered the virey, the deeper grew the hatred of the Spaniards against him. Their acts of violence and their cruelty were prompted by their greed for gold. Their sole purpose for coming to America, was to grow rich quickly, and they could only expect to succeed in this, if they could force the peaceable Indians to serve them in the attainment of this object.

It was seldom that one of the earlier vireys of Peru had been guided by humane principles in his government, as a rule, they were no better than the fortune-hunters, who flocked to this land of promise.

Cinchon was a man of a different character. He was a Christian with all his heart and soul, and therefore full of mercy and love for his fellow-beings. This fundamental trait of his character showed itself in all his measures, and prompted the formulating of the laws, which he issued by virtue of his power. It is true, that in the first years of his administration, this did not show itself so much, because he was not yet thoroughly acquainted with conditions as they really were. It thus happened that he was much beloved in Lima because of his mild rule. The peace, which the city of Lima, and in fact, all the Spanish settlements enjoyed since his coming, and the firmness with which the late insurrection of the Indians had been quelled, all deepened this regard for the virey, which found such a generous expression in the ovations brought him after his recovery. But now he learned the true state of affairs, through the trustworthy descriptions of Huahamac. With characteristic energy he at once set about to devise means for the relief of the shamefully oppressed nation. It had always been the custom to slander unpopular vireys at the court of Madrid. This was the more easy, because the king of Spain very reluctantly placed his power in the new world, in the hands of a virey, and consequently was mistrustful and jealous to a marked degree. Whether the charges brought were purely invented or not, he never took the time to investigate. But if at any time there was an investigation, it was entrusted to some individual, whose position entitled him to the succession in the office, so that it was most natural to find the charges sustained. There was no other way for such an individual to attain his desired object, namely to sit in the virey's place. And the favor of the fickle people ever turned to the new ruler.

This plan had been tried too often since the days of Pizarro, not to suggest itself now. The virey had shown himself as a friend of the Indians, and the favor of the people turned from him, nay was changed into its very opposite.

The citizens of Lima had a natural inclination for plotting and conspiring, and they did not hesitate an instant to use every means to stop the virey's plan. They seemed to be convinced that if he continued along his lines, in a few years, instead of being benefitted and enriched, they would be empoverished and destroyed.

This was enough to cause them to cast their full hatred upon Don Cinchon.

And so these lying accusations, these slanders against the virey were sent to Spain. The weightiest charge against him was, that he favored the Indians because they had bribed him, having brought him immeasurable wealth in gold. They said, that he considered only his own advantage; that he was as severe with the Spaniards, as he was lenient with the Indians. They intimated that his plan was, with the aid of the Indians, to make himself independent of Spain as ruler of Peru.

Thus the seeds of distrust and jealousy were sown at the court of the king of Spain, and the accursed seed fell upon a ground very favorable to the slanderers. In Spain they did not dare to proceed against the virey in the manner which had been customary since the days of Columbus, the discoverer of America, for they had to consider his high position, and his powerful and wealthy family. Every ship arriving from Callao however, brought fresh reports, until there appeared to be sufficient material upon which to base a serious charge against Cinchon. They were only too ready and willing at the court of Madrid, to receive these accusations, which were constantly arriving from Lima, as pure, unadulterated truth. However, in order at least to preserve the appearance of justice, the whole case against the virey of Peru was referred to the Castilian tribunal for careful investigation. This was a course of proceedure, which invariably led to the result desired by the king. They never thought of asking the virey to answer the charges brought against him, or if it was thought of, they never considered it worth while to act accordingly. The verdict against him was formulated; he was to be recalled, and only upon his arrival at Madrid was he once more to be tried before a tribunal of justice.

However, the tremendous distance separating Lima and Madrid, and the long time required by the slow-sailing vessels of that day to make the trip, caused years to pass before the charges were in, and the verdict rendered, and finally published at Lima. The virey had no intimation of what had been so treacherously plotted against him. Actuated by the dictates of his noble heart, he continued along the course he had set himself to follow. Without the least consideration for the name or the station of the offenders; whoever was guilty of violence against the Indians, was delivered over to the punishment prescribed by the law. By such strict measures he called down upon himself the hatred of those whom he had punished, while he lost the last bit of favor with the people. This change of public feeling began soon after his recovery. It was carefully kept from him however, and all the more certain he fell into the pit which had been dug for him.

Popular favor is a most uncertain thing, and no age forms an exception in this particular. Who would' ever have believed that the people would so soon have tried every means to destroy that man, whom they had brought such grand ovations upon his first visit to the cathedral after his convalescence?

The problem is simply and easily solved. With those laws which Cinchon had enacted for the protection of the Indians, he touched the selfishness of his people, indeed he touched their very hearts. But it is one of the sadest experiences of life, that the so-called good friendships among men find their deepest roots and their limits as well in selfishness. As long as you extend certain privileges and advantages to a man, he is your friend; but the moment these privileges are withdrawn, his friendship for you not only will cease, but somehow he gets an idea, that these advantages are being purposely withheld, and a bitter hatred and enmity may take the place of his former friendship. This is a common experience, and has been a cause for complaint in all times.

This is what Cinchon now had to experience. The Spaniards had been highly pleased at the peace, whose blessings they enjoyed, at the security they felt since the Indians had been so completely conquered, and now humbly bowed before their victors. At first they were inclined to overlook the virey's exceptionally favorable attitude toward the Indians, because of the advantages which they enjoyed, and because he was very lenient with them also, and showed no trace of that haughty spirit, which demanded of everyone to bow low before him, because the virey was to Peru, what the king was to Spain.

But all the sharper was their change of feeling toward him after his recovery, when it became apparent that he not only had firmly decided to break the Spaniards of their brutality against the natives, but showed openly his friendship for the Indians, whom he offered advantages upon every occasion. Those who held influential positions in Lima were soon filled with bitter hatred, and they were followed by the subordinate officials. They were joined by the monks of the mission stations, who also had to sacrifice many privileges which they had formerly enjoyed, and who well knew that the cause for the changed conditions lay with Cinchon.

This hatred not only fell upon the virey, but also upon Huahamac. It was believed that to his friendly intercourse with the virey, the latter's favorable attitude toward the Indians was to be attributed. It was also believed, that from the chief the virey learned of the acts of violence perpetrated by individual Spaniards upon the Indians. The more Huahamac was honored and beloved by his people, who well knew what they owed him, the deeper grew the hatred of the Spaniards against him They did not dare to get their revenge openly, because they feared the vindictive hatred of the Indians, and so they sought secret ways of getting their satisfaction, which brought them success more surely than Huahamac would have dreamed.

Perhaps jealousy is nowhere to be found to a greater degree than among the serving class. The favor, real or imaginary, shown one before the others, is ground for bitter hatred, whose source is envy.

The relation of Hualma to Dolores was sisterly, toward the virey it was that of a child. This aroused envy and hatred with the servants of the virey's household. They saw in her only the Indian. That reverence of the Peruvians for one in whose veins ran the blood of the Incas, who was a member of the ruling family, found no place in the soul of a negro from Africa. And this enmity eventually delivered her over into the hands of Cinchon's enemies.

With jealous eyes they regarded Hualma, to whom they would concede only the condition of slavery, so long as she abode in Lima as an hostage. The higher she rose in the estimation of the virey and his daughter, the deeper grew the hatred against her. The "duenna" already advanced in years, was not proof against this. As the love of Dolores for Hualma deepened, she felt her influence wane, and her heart turned away from Hualma to the slaves. The "duenna" knew the legend of the Indians concerning the remedy for the fever. She knew of the solemn oath of the Indians, for she was the most confidential servant of the virey's family. It is possible also, that she played eavesdropper, when Huahamac and the virey met after the latter's convalescence. She would not have considered that a wrong against her enemy. At any rate, she openly declared, and quite positively too, that

Hualma must have received the remedy from her father, whose extraordinary effect was the cause of the recovery of the virey and his daughter Dolores. With this statement there agreed what was told by one of the negroes, who said, that on the night preceding the remarkable improvement in the condition of the patients, he had seen Huahamac secretly enter the palace, hand a small parcel to Hualma, and then disappear again.

There was not an individual in the servant's hall of the palace, who had any doubt whatever, but that Huahamac had broken the Indians' oath. These secret enemies of Hualma knew perfectly well, that they could not undertake anything against her personally, but the hateful old Spanish "duenna" conceived a diabolical plan. She would drive a sword into the soul of the girl, by the almost certain murder of her father by the Indians. This was to be her revenge, because she imagined that Hualma had crowded her out of her place of intimacy with Dolores. Her vile plan was at once put into operation. Through the Indians who regularly came to Lima to market, she hoped to scatter the seeds of hatred against Huahamac among the people of his tribe, dwelling in the heart of the distant mountains. The negroes were at once ready to serve the old woman with all their trickery and treachery, for they were anxious to destroy Hualma, whom in their envy they hated, although she had never harmed one of them.

The plan pursued by these plotters was far-reaching, but sure. Count Cinchon's negroes knew how to put themselves into communication with the Indians. In the most harmless manner they related to them as if it had been a fact, the story they had so artfully put together, and its effects was all the more sure. Thus there gathered a dangerous cloud over the head of Huahamac, of which he had not the least intimation, and at the same time one of the best viceroys of Peru was in danger of being undone. Although the persecution of these two was being pursued independently by the enemies of each, it really sprang from the same root. The secret slander against Cinchon took a longer time to accomplish its end, because it had to make use of various channels, because the distance between Peru and Spain was so great, and the means of communication so scant. On the other hand the plot against Huahamac promised to develop much more quickly, and actually did. But as the hand of the Almighty is everywhere the surest and safest protection, so it was evidently over Huahamac, who was to be the instrument through which God planned to bestow infinite blessings upon men, both here and beyond the seas.

CHAPTER VII.

It was an easy matter to enter into communication with the Indians who daily brought fruit to the market at Lima, and the negroes together with their friends and accomplices, did not delay putting the "duenna's" plan into operation. At first the Indians seemed to pay little attention to the gossip of the negroes, but when they repeated the story at home, a different face was put upon the matter. Long since it had been suspected, that Huahamac inclined to the religion of the Spaniards as Hualma had done, who became a Christian. The frequent visits to the virey, and more still his constant visits to the mission, confirmed this suspicion. This was reason sufficient for the priests to give credence to the story, which the Indians, who had been to market, brought home from Lima. They were shrewd enough not to confide to the Indians their opinions, but whenever an opportunity afforded, they communicated the story to the tribal chiefs.

A secret meeting of the chiefs and priests was thereupon held. Breaking the oath was a crime among the Indians, which brought certain death; but in the eyes of his people, Huahamac was a sacred person. He belonged to the few descendants of the Incas, was the oldest of them in fact, and in the eyes of the Indians, undisputed ruler of all Peru, to whom all were subject. They certainly could not be careless in dealing with so grave an accusation in his case. They therefore determined, first of all to carefully investigate, and if sufficient evidence were found to warrant it, to call Huahamac to account. In their natural devotion to the Inca, the people refused to believe the charge of the priests, whom they knew to be greedy for power, and they resented the way in which their chief was being attacked. On the other hand the priests did not give up their plan to destroy Huahamac. They had a deep-rooted suspicion of his faithlessness toward the religion of his people. This was the ground of their hatred.

Huahamac learned nothing of the hostile plans, — — — at least, so his adversaries thought; but their plan, like so many founded on absolute secrecy, was not so sure as they imagined.

An Indian, the son of a chief, had grown up with Huahamac, who had lost his parents early, during a persecution by the Spaniards. This man was supposed to succeed his father as chieftain.

Between Huahamac and this Indian there existed a deep friendship, which up to this time, had stood every test, and never been dimmed. The old chief was still living, but he had become childish from age, and his son, Huahamac's friend, while not yet actually chief of his tribe, represented his father in the councils.

He was much disturbed by the charge against Huahamac. He alone thoroughly knew the Inca. He knew better than any of them, of what things Huahamac was capable, when his fidelity was put to the test. Once he had been wounded unto death in a battle with the Spaniards, and Huahamac had saved his life, by carrying the wounded man for miles upon his shoulders, far into the safety of the mountains, until exhausted, he fell in a faint, where other Indians found them. That experience this true and faithful man had not forgotten, for his grateful heart would not permit it. When he thought of Huahamac's love for his child, for the virey, and for the Donna Dolores, he knew that for these he would be capable of bringing any sacrifice. When therefore, he learned in the secret council, that the virey and Dolores had lain at death's door, and when he recalled what Huahamac had said to him about the oath of the Indians, it became clear to his mind, that the Inca had done from motives of pure love, that thing of which he was accused. He wisely kept these thoughts to himself however, and determined to speak with Huahamac, and if it were true, then he would do by him, as Huahamac had done by him years ago, when he had saved his life.

A few weeks later Huahamac was sitting before the door of his hut, enjoying the delightful coolness of a mild evening. The evening breezes wafted over to him marvellous perfumes from the blossoming trees and shrubs of the nearlying hills. The little brook, which ran into the valley over a steep incline just opposite his hut, sang its song, and with it were mingled the voices of the birds awakening to new life, after the moderating of the intense heat of the day. Half dreaming, half waking, his thoughts were busy with his beloved child, who unfortunately, was compelled still to remain in Lima by the provisions of the treaty of peace.

Suddenly he heard the leaves softly rustling by his side. Only the ear of an Indian could have detected the sound. Huahamac drew himself up. His hand seized the tomahawk. In those times no Indian was without his tomahawk at any time, for he was never safe from the bitter persecutions of the Spaniards. At the same instant he observed an Indian who, having come out of the woods, soon stood before him. It was his foster-brother.

"Just let your tomahawk rest," said the Indian with a smile as he drew near. Huahamac again quietly lay down upon the soft moss, and a few moments later the Indian lay beside him.

"Huahamac," said he, "do you remember how you carried me out of the thick of the battle, and regardless of your own danger, saved my life?"

"Those are things of the past," replied Huahamac, "one ought not to speak of them any longer."

"But they ought not to be forgotten either," returned the other, "so that one may not forget what is due the friend, when the time has come to make return."

Huahamac raised himself quickly. His penetrating glance fixed itself upon the face of the Indian.

"What do these words mean?" he asked, "I am not on the war path, and neither are you."

"There are paths much more dangerous than the warpath," said the Indian. "Upon the warpath you are able to defend yourself against your enemy. This you can not do when a treacherous snake uncoils itself behind you, without your seeing it, in order to bury its fangs in your body."

"I see no venomous serpent," cried Huahamac in astonishment.

"Perhaps it is all the more dangerous for that reason," returned his friend.

"But I do not understand you, my brother! Speak plainly, that I may know what kind of an enemy you mean," said Huahamac.

"You frequently go to the missions," said the Indian.

"It is true," was Huahamac's brief reply.

"You are being watched," continued his friend.

"I know it," said Huahamac with a disdainful curl of his lip.

"They are watching you, and suspect you of falling away from the faith of the fathers. Hualma, your child, a daughter of the Incas, has already done this thing," continued the Indian.

"And did not Huascar, a son of the Incas, do the same thing before her?" asked Huahamac.

"He did, and he became estranged from his people. You are the rightful head of our nation. Do you consider, why you are watched, why suspicions have been aroused, and why they are beginning to mistrust you?" said the Indian in a low tone.

Huahamac remained silent for a time, as if in deep thought.

"Since when is it forbidden an Inca to investigate the teachings of another people? To whom is he account-able for this?" he said quietly but firmly.

"To no one, Huahamac, my brother," answered the Indian, lowering his head; "but the priests demand of an Inca, the head of the nation, that he be true to the faith of the fathers. This can not be unknown to you."

"Are you saying these things of yourself?" asked Huahamac pointedly. "Is this your opinion also?"

"Yes, and no, as you will have it," replied his friend. "I tell you this, because my love for you prompts me to speak openly to you. I tell you also, however, because the priests have held a meeting of the tribal chiefs, in which they charged you with this thing. You must know the plans of your opponents, I will not call them enemies."

Huahamac leaped to his feet excitedly. In his hand he clenched his tomahawk. His eyes flashed in hot anger.

"You called and held a meeting without me? You took counsel without me, and without hearing me?" he cried in angry excitement.

"It was done," calmly answered the Indian, "because another grave accusation was raised against you, a charge which I scarcely dare to mention, because its truth would arm the hands of your opponents against you, openly and secretly. Your life would be forfeited for breaking faith, and for breaking our solemn oath."

The Indian looked at him sharply as he said this, yet, even though the consciousness of his guilt made his heart beat faster for a moment, the keen eye of the Indian could discover no trace of emotion in Huahamac's face.

"Speak out," said Huahamac with a firm voice.

"It is claimed," said the Indian, that you brought our secret remedy to the virey and his daughter, or rather that you gave it to your daughter Hualma, and by its use, both of them, already at the verge of the grave, were healed in a wonderful manner."

"Who says that?" asked Huahamac in an almost careless tone.

"The priests," replied the Indian.

"And what is the source of their information?" asked Huahamac in the same careless tone.

"One of the black slaves of the virey claims, that he saw you secretly enter the palace under the cover of darkness, and go to the apartment of your daughter, to whom you gave a package. He says, that you gave Hualma careful instructions concerning the use of the medicine, and on the following day the patients showed a marked improvement."

Huahamac was silent a moment, then he proudly raised his head.

"If a man were convinced of the right of his action, would the oath forbid giving the remedy to a Spaniard, or does it forbid revealing its nature and the source whence it is obtained?" he asked.

The Indian was evidently surprised by the question. He stared at the ground before him and remained silent for a long time. He carefully proved the oath which he also had sworn, and after a calm consideration of the matter, he came to the conclusion, that the oath merely forbade revealing the nature of the remedy to the Spaniards, but it said nothing about giving the powder, so long as its nature remained a secret. His better knowledge and his conscience compelled the Indian to give a negative answer to the question. An expression of great joy came over his face. Leaping to his feet, he cried:

"No, Huahamac, no, the oath does not speak of that."

"Come along then," said the Inca, "let us call a council of the chiefs."

"You are right," replied the Indian. As night began to fall, the two were seen entering the forest with hasty strides.

Three days later the chiefs were assembled about their head priest. A gigantic magnolia stood in the middle of their place of meeting, among whose dark, glossy leaves hung the rosy fruit, giving the tree a most beautiful appearance.

Against its smooth trunk, leaned Huahamac, the Inca.

His bow was slung over his shoulder, and upon his back hung the quiver, made of the fibres of the palm. In his right hand he held a large, magnificently ornamented tomahawk, while his left grasped a half dozen light, slender spears. Upon his head he wore a gaudy crown of parrot-feathers.

He was tall in stature, perfect in proportion, and extraordinarily muscular. The color of his skin was much lighter than that of the other Peruvians, and this color, approaching that of the Spaniards, was the unmistakable sign of his descent from the Incas. The expression of his face was earnest, nay almost forbidding. His bushy eyebrows were drawn together, and from under them his eyes flashed forth, bringing almost a terror to the hearts of some upon whom his piercing glance fell. All the chiefs had answered the call. Silently they sat at the feet of the man, to whom they all conceded the right to rule over them.

At length Huahamac raised himself to his full height with as much pride in his manner, as natural dignity. His flashing eyes swept around the circle of expectant chiefs and priests. Then he began to speak, and his voice sounded like the deep roll of distant thunder, but the longer he spoke, the richer and fuller it grew. In the sharpest terms he rebuked them for having broken the custom of their people, the hallowed usage since time immemorial, in that they had dared to call and hold a council against, and without the knowledge of the Inca. His words fell like bolts of lightning. They lowered their eyes before him, and even the priests felt, that the sword of vengeance hung over them by a hair. With inward satisfaction Huahamac noted the effect of his words.

Without pronouncing any further judgment excepting the severest condemnation of their action. for which he also sharply rebuked them, he proceeded to take up the second point, that they had dared to sit in judgment over him without giving him the least opportunity to defend himself.

His words fell heavily upon the men sitting around in the circle. Shame and the consciousness, that they had deserved such chiding, nay crushing words, were written upon every face. Everyone keenly felt how completely Huahamac had the right on his side.

He was silent for a few moments, then in somewhat higher tone which he gradually lowered as he proceeded, he expressed his deep contempt, because they had caused his steps to be watched by spies. This struck home with the priests. With an expression of profound grief he asked:

"Since when is the Inca of Peru deprived of his freedom? Since when is it commanded that a father's heart is to be closed against love for his child?"

As he said this his voice trembled. The effect was most stirring. All eyes were fixed upon the man, whose life and deeds appeared spotless before them, and in these eyes he read approval.

Suddenly he raised his voice to its full power, and stepping into the centre of the circle he cried:

"Stand forth, ye enemies of mine, ye who charge me with gravest fault of all, with having broken the oath! Stand forth, and freely and openly say whereof ye have secretly accused me to the chiefs!"

He laid down his bow, the quiver, spears and tomahawk in the circle, and taking off his crown of feathers, placed it upon them. Then he cried with a voice of thunder:

"Come forth, come forth with your charge that I have broken the oath! Here I have laid down the symbols of my honor, and I shall not touch them again, if I am found guilty."

The priests trembled, fearing to look into his face, but not one of them moved. As if by magic, however, all the chiefs leaped to their feet and cried:

"Take up again the hallowed symbols of your honorable office. We are not your judges, but you are ours. Hail to the Inca Huahamac. Death and destruction to all slanderous tongues!"

Each one of the tribal chiefs made haste to seize one of the articles laid aside by Huahamac, and approaching him, to offer it to him.

For a time Huahamac hesitated, then however, he again received the weapons and the crown of feathers, and with a firm voice he said:

"Very well then, I will do as you request."

"Render judgment!" cried the chiefs deeply moved.

"No," said Huahamac, "no. The stain is not yet removed from me, even though they lack the courage to tell me to my face, what they charged me with in secret, I shall do it myself. Hear me!"

He again stepped back under the leafy roof of the magnolia, under which he had been standing at the opening of the council. He began to tell them of all the kindness and affection which the noble virey and Donna Dolores had bestowed upon his daughter Hualma, who, although she had accepted the faith of the Christians, was nevertheless his only child, the treasure of his soul. He described the violent illness which had seized upon them both, and showed them how they must inevitably have died of the fever. He placed before them the manner of the virey, and laid stress upon the duty of gratefulness toward the man who had proved himself ever a friend of the Indians, and their greatest benefactor. He pictured the noble soul of the man with an enthusiasm, which deeply moved the hearts of the listeners. He then pointed out, that if Cinchon had died, probably another one of those inhuman rulers would have come to Peru, of whom so many had preceded him, since the "Children of the Sun", as the Peruvians called the Spaniards, had first come sailing across the salt water to the shores of Peru. He described with much feeling the scene, when Hualma had knelt before him, and implored him to give her the remedy, of which she herself was ignorant.

Then, he continued, he had carefully proven the oath which he, which they all had sworn. He found that the oath required nothing more, than that no one of his people should reveal the remedy to the Spaniards, that no one should show them the tree whose bark furnished it; that no one should reveal to them the place where it struck its roots into the earth. Not one word was said however, by which it was forbidden to give the self-prepared powder to a Spaniard, who, by his kindness to the Indians, had merited it, in order to save him from certain death. When he had gained this conviction, after severe inner conflicts, he had gone into the mountains and had peeled off some of the bark of the sacred trees of Pachicamak. He had dried the bark and ground it to powder, which he brought to Hualma, who was overjoyed to receive it. He had also given her some instructions as to the manner in which the brownish powder was to be administered. He had thereby preserved the benefactor, nay the father of the Peruvian people, and for Hualma a loving sister.

"This is my wrong, if it be one; this is the breaking of the oath with which I have been charged. Not one, not my dear Hualma, nor the noble virey, nor his child, knows what the remedy is, nor where it can be found. I have preserved a fatherly heart for my people. This is my fault."

He was silent and looked around the circle. Again all the chiefs leaped to their feet crying:

"Hail, hail to the Inca Huahamac! Death to the slanderers!"

"No!" cried Huahamac. "I know that jealousy and envy of my dear child, who enjoys the confidence and love of Donna Dolores; I know that jealousy and envy of me, among those who are in the palace of the virey, have determined to destroy both my daughter and me. They were very shrewd in selecting the method by which to secure belief for their lies. Unfortunately they found open ears and hearts, which were not friendly disposed toward me. I will judge as my heart dictates. I forgive all who have done me wrong."

He was about to turn and leave the council, but the priests approached, and throwing themselves down at his feet, they implored:

"Noble Inca, forgive!"

"I have forgiven you," said he, and turning away, he left the meeting. From a distance, however, he heard the cries of approval and the praise of his name. That night he slept in his hut, and calmer than for many months.

CHAPTER VIII.

Huahamac was in doubt a long time, whether to tell the virey, or his daughter Hualma, anything about his experiences; however, Hualma occasionally came in contact with Peruvians, with whom she was accustomed to speak in her dearly beloved mother tongue. In this way she found out all about the occurence. At first she was greatly disturbed by the matter, but her fears were allayed by the fortunate outcome. Then she related all the circumstances to Dolores, and was happy because the virey's daughter highly praised her father's action.

Thus everything came to the ears of Count Cinchon also. When Huahamac came to the palace shortly after, the virey drew him into his private room and had a long audience with him. Huahamac could not refrain from revealing to Cinchon the · trickery whereby the old "duenna", and the negroes in the virey's employ, had hoped to destroy him and his daughter Hualma.

The soul of a man like Cinchon must be filled with deepest loathing by such base treachery. Huahamac earnestly begged him not to follow up this revelation of the plot against him and Hualma, because the serpent had been made harmless by the breaking out of its poisonous fang; but the virey felt that he could not conscientiously permit the matter to pass over unnoticed. At first he was inclined to send the treacherous old creature back to Spain by the first vessel leaving Callao; but Dolores begged so warmly for mercy for her "duenna", who was otherwise most faithful, and sincerely devoted to her, that he gave up this idea.

The culprit did not, however, escape all punishment. The virey summoned her and called her to a severe account. She recognized then the wrong she had done, and frankly acknowledged it, showing sincere repentance. And so the old relations between her and the family were reestablished, indeed, the old "duenna" became the instrument, whereby Cinchon's eyes were opened to the treachery planned against him.

Dolores had but little intercourse with the ladies of the aristocratic families of Lima, the "duenna" however.

cultivated the acquaintance of a great number of women belonging to the middle class, who stood nearer her station. She frequently called upon them, and they often visited her. There was always, of course, a great deal of gossip. One of these women, who entertained a particular liking for Dolores, during a visit spoke about the feeling of animosity to the virey, of which she had learned through her husband.

The "duenna" grew attentive. She began to question about the matter, and her talkative friend told her everything she knew about it. But this was enough to reveal the whole dastardly scheme, in which high and low were involved, and to show its motive and ultimate object.

It is true, the anger of the virey had deeply humiliated the old "duenna", for she had grown up in his family, and had carried him in her arms, just as later she had carried his daughter Dolores. She was all the more happy to show him a service now, whereby she would again gain his favor and confidence. With breathless haste she returned to the palace. She alone had the privilege to enter the virey's apartments unannounced, and so she went directly to him. She found him in earnest conversation with Huahamac.

The presence of the Indian disturbed her.

The virey knew the old woman too well, not to see from the anxiety written upon her face and from her excited manner, that she had something of grave importance to communicate to him.

"Stay here," said he kindly to her; "you can speak freely before this man, no matter what it may be that you have to tell me."

She approached and began to tell all she knew.

The virey listened to her with increasing interest.

Huahamac was more disturbed by the things he heard than Cinchon

"Wretched people!" cried he, "which is innocently compelled to furnish weapons against the man, whom it praises as its greatest benefactor!"

"Do not say that, Huahamac," said the virey deeply moved. "How can your unfortunate people be blamed, if the wild passions of my countrymen cause them to blame me for my gentleness and benevolence? How can they be blamed, if my countrymen seek by lying and deceit to destroy me, as if I had been injurious to their best interests? Did they act any differently toward my predecessors?"

"But what are you going to do?" asked Huahamac. "What course are you going to pursue in order to wrest the tomahawk from the hands of your enemies? What plan do you propose to follow in order to secure a clear trail for justice and right?"

The virey sat thinking for a while, then he calmly said:

"There are only three ways open. Either I must quietly await the result, or I must write a justification to free myself of all the charges they have brought against me, or, finally, I must sail at once, in order to go to the king in person, and reveal the network of treachery against me."

"If I were permitted to counsel you," said Huahamac modestly, "I would advise you to choose the last course. It is the surest, and the only one to lead you directly to the goal. And I, I shall hasten to my people and call a council, so that as a representative I may accompany you, in order to testify in the name of the Peruvians, to your dealings, and to bear witness to your high and noble spirit."

The virey looked upon the Inca with deep emotion. Then he seized his hand and pressed it warmly.

"I thank you, Huahamac," said he. "This expression of your fidelity to me but strengthens the bond of friendship already existing between us. But I must calmly and carefully consider all things before acting. Stay here, or come again to-morrow. By that time I will have reached a positive decision."

"Not tomorrow," said Huahamac. "Give me three days. They will not matter much."

The virey agreed to this. The Indian hastened back to his mountains, while the virey sent a mounted messenger to the captain of a vessel, lying ready to sail in the harbor of Callao, in order to detain him, until he should have come to a definite conclusion concerning his course of action.

Huahamac had scarcely reached the home of the nearest chief, when he sent messengers in every direction, in order to call the people to a great council at the well-known meeting-place, under the huge magnolia. From tribe to tribe flew the messengers of the Inca. On the following morning already, great crowds of armed Indians could be seen taking their way from the mountains, out of the passes and valleys, and encamping in the familiar place of meeting. By noon Huahamac was justified in considering the council full and could formally open the meeting with his address.

His address was remarkable for its simplicity, clearness and warmth. He explained the situation to the assembly, and reminded them of the obligations they had over against the virey, and that their gratefulness to him should urge them to bear testimony to the truth. He then declared his intention of accompanying the virey across the big saltwater, if his people should choose to delegate him. He would endeavor to clear their benefactor of the stain, which his enemies had tried to fix upon him. As with

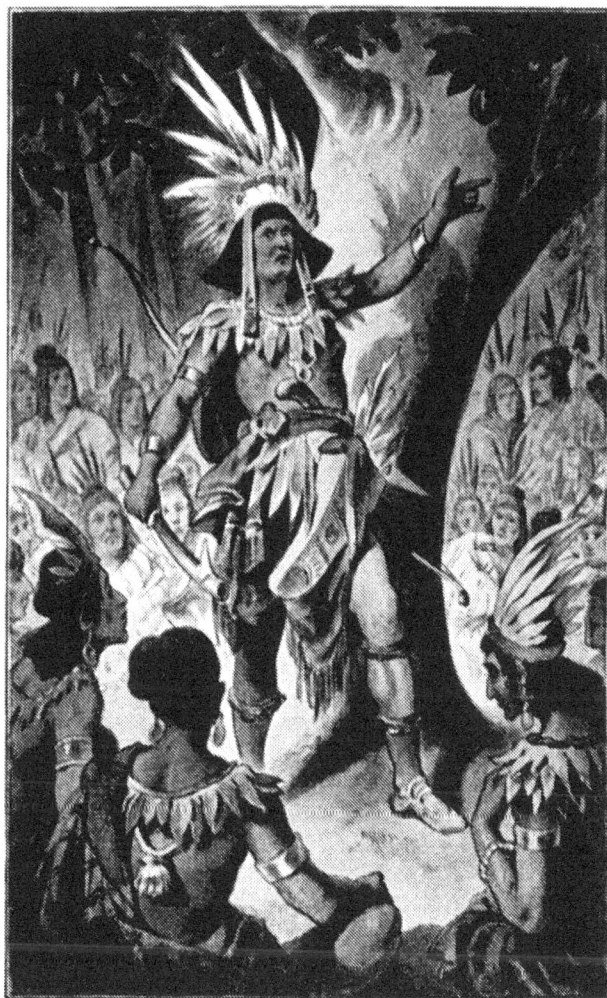

one voice, the numerous assembly gave their assent. Huahamac had not miscalculated.

In the meantime, the resolution had become fixed in the soul of the virey, to prevent his enemies. He had communicated his intentions to Dolores, and given her the choice, either to remain in Lima until he should return, or to accompany him to Spain. Dolores soon reached her decision. She declared, that under no circumstances would she permit herself to be separated from her beloved father. Hualma was present during this interview between Cinchon and his daughter. She was deeply affected by what she heard and saw, and when Dolores asked her what she would do in the matter, she arose, and placing her hand on her heart, she said:

"Can the earth want the light, without being in darkness? Can the earth lack the quickening and nurturing sunlight, without becoming cold and dead? Where thou goest, Hualma will follow, and be it into death."

Dolores embraced her, with tears in her eyes, and the virey kissed her forehead, as he said:

"Thou most faithful friend!"

The most necessary preparations were now made for the hasty departure. When evening came, Huahamac appeared in the full dress of a Peruvian Inca.

"I come with the full authority of an envoy of the people of Peru to the king across the great salt-water," he said with dignity. "My mission is to bear testimony to the faithfulness and uprightness of the virey. How is it, must I make the long voyage alone?"

"No, my dear friend," answered the virey, heartily shaking his hand. "To-night we sail together."

"But Hualma will accompany us?" Huahamac asked. "I need her as my interpreter, since I can but poorly speak your native tongue, while she uses it perfectly."

"Hualma will accompany us," answered the virey, "because she will not be separated from Dolores. Go to her, so that you may be convinced that it is her own free decision."

Don Perez was announced. He was the most liberal of the Spaniards in his position over against the Peruvians, and the virey had therefore selected him as his representative during his absence. He placed the appointment in his hands, and recommended the Peruvians to his kind consideration.

Perez, as well as the whole city of Lima, were suprised at the sudden, unexpected departure of the virey. No decision had as yet been received from the court at Madrid, and yet he sailed for home. Perez, moreover, had nothing to do with the intrigues against Cinchon, indeed they were unknown to him, because he was numbered with the friends of the virey.

With great astonishment he learned the circumstances from Cinchon's lips. He quickly determined to draw up a true and honest statement of the facts, before the virey's departure, and therefore asked him to put it off until the following morning. To this Don Cinchon consented. Perez then hastened to carry out what his honest, open soldier-heart had prompted him to do.

A mounted messenger brought the document to the virey, just as the vessel in which he, Huahamac, Dolores and Hualma had taken passage, was about to sail. A favorable wind filled the sails, the prow was turned to the open sea. A few hours sailing sufficed to withdraw from view the mountains of blood-saturated Peru.

CHAPTER IX.

Seldom was the dangerous voyage Cinchon had undertaken, completed with so little discomfort. There was not even a mishap.

With a certain feeling of uneasiness, the usually brave Huahamac and his daughter Hualma, had gone aboard the frail vessel. This feeling lingered with them for quite a while, and grew stronger when land was lost to view. On the open sea they became conscious, more than ever before, of the helplessness and feebleness of man. This was a most favorable opportunity to show them the blessedness of the Christian faith, which fills the heart of man with confidence toward God. Dolores discharged this office of Christian love toward Hualma, while the earnest, deeply pious virey did the same toward Huahamac. An aged missionary, who had faithfully served his Master among the Indians of Peru, was returning to Spain, to spend the declining years of his life in well-deserved rest. He thoroughly understood the Peruvian language, and completed the holy work. Never had he found a pupil more eager to learn the teachings of Jesus, who received them with greater clearness of understanding or with more earnestness, or who was better prepared, than Huahamac.

Bonifacio daily devoted himself to his holy task of instructing his pupil, and one day, as they were nearing the coast of Spain, Huahamac said to him:

"Dear Father, give me, I pray you, the seal of communion with Jesus Christ, the blessed sacrament of Baptism, so that I may enter the land of the Christians as a Christian."

Highly pleased with the request of the Inca, the

priest consented. Huahamac's knowledge was sufficient, his faith was strong and joyous. The solemn ceremony took place on the deck of the vessel, which, swimming on the deep, formed a strange baptistry. No one was more happy over the event, than Hualma, and her dear friend and sister Dolores. The relation between Huahamac and Don Cinchon grew more intimate still from this time on. The Indian and his child were no longer strangers, they were members of the count's family.

A new world was opened to Huahamac and Hualma when they landed on the shores of Spain. Everything they saw appeared strange, new and wonderful to them. They received these new impressions in silence, and only when alone with Don Cinchon and Dolores, a thousand questions were asked, which the virey and his daughter cheerfully answered.

Don Cinchon had reported his arrival, and that of the Inca of Peru, immediately upon landing. He was notified, that he was to wait in a city near the capital, until he should receive the summons to appear at court. This showed him that the slanderous reports of his enemies had been only too readily received. In the consciousness of his innocence, he willingly submitted to every arrangement, even though frequently his soul was deeply hurt.

Nevertheless all the honors due to his office, were shown him. The summons to appear at court was long delayed. Suddenly however, there came a change. As cool as they had formerly been toward him, so warm and friendly they now showed themselves. Don Cinchon could not understand this sudden change, and yet the explanation was very simple.

Father Bonifacio, although he had never spoken with the virey about the matter, was yet fully informed about the troubles that compelled him to make the long voyage to Spain. He knew perfectly the conditions prevailing in Lima, and some things which had been dark to him, were cleared up by his conversations with Huahamac. Knowing what he did, he felt himself compelled to speak a word in favor of the much slandered virey. He had learned to know him well during the long voyage, and had come to esteem and love him.

As soon as the prior of the cloister to which he belonged gave him permission, he hastened to Madrid. It was not a difficult matter for him to secure an introduction at court. Here he gave his testimony as truthfully, as it was strong and emphatic. This produced a profound effect. He had to remain upon command of the king, in order to repeat his testimony before the Castilian tribunal of justice. In the meantime the report of Don Perez was received, which was found to correspond almost literally with the statements of Father Bonifacio. The slander and treachery of Cinchon's enemies were thus unmasked. Father Bonifacio also strongly advocated Cinchon's method of dealing with the Indians. He also claimed that only a mild and gentle treatment of them would secure a firm foundation for Spanish rule in Peru. The greed for gold and the cruelty of the Spaniards living there, and of those who kept coming, would have to be controlled, if this object was to be attained, and as well a higher object, namely the conversion of the Peruvians to Christianity. From his own long experience he showed how the cruel treatment of the Indians by the Spaniards, had crippled the work of the Christian missions for a long time to come. They could only succeed if the government would go hand in hand with Don Cinchon and the missionaries in their efforts.

He gave the same advice before the Castilian council, which had already received the report of Don Perez. These two testimonies thoroughly unsettled their preconceived opinions. The sentence which had already been rendered, was revoked, and with one stroke the whole situation was changed. Don Cinchon was now summoned to appear at court. All the honors due his office, were lavishly bestowed upon him, and wherever he appeared Donna Dolores shared his honors with him. The presence of the virey at court, was celebrated with great pomp. The king with his own hand hung about his neck the highest decoration of Spain, the order of the golden fleece. Although Cinchon and Huahamac both demanded a hearing in the matter against the virey, no one would consider such a request.

Everyone wondered at the noble bearing of the Inca. He was highly honored, and received many valuable gifts from all sides. Hualma also soon became the favorite of the queen, and thereby, as is usually the case, of the whole court. Feast followed feast, honors followed upon honors at the court of Madrid for a full three months.

One day, as they were sitting quietly together, Huahamac said to his friend, the virey:

"I am weary of this intoxicating life at court. It robs me of my peace and health. More and more a yearning for the mountains and the woods of my home is growing upon me. Verily, I prefer my humble cabin amid the lofty mountains of Peru, to the royal palace. What I have here seen and learned shall be of benefit to my people. I will tell them, that it is foolishness to war against your nation. Wars will only lessen our number, and blood will be needlessly and uselessly spilt. The only road to blessing and fortune is, to go hand in hand with you, to learn to know and to pray to your God, to leave forever the warpath, and to learn from you the arts of peace."

He stopped suddenly. Then he turned his eye full upon Don Cinchon.

"But you, will you return to the land where you were treated so ungratefully by your own countrymen?" he asked. "Sometimes I have doubted it. I beg of you, I entreat you, return with me. You brought us blessings unnumbered, you will keep them for us."

"Under one condition, I will return," said Don Cinchon smilingly, as he seized Huahamac's hand. "Under the condition that you and your people will reveal to us the remedy for the fever. You will do a great work, you will do a deed blessed among men and worthy before God, if you will persuade your people "

Huahamac agreed.

"I am a Christian," he said firmly, "and that oath which I swore, was a sin before God. It no longer binds me, and even though my people should refuse their consent, I will teach you and your people to know the healing tree. This I promise you before the face of Him, who is your Lord and mine, your God and Judge and mine. Amen."

About a year and a half later a vessel appeared in the harbor of Callao, flying the standard of the king of Spain. The commandant of the harbor of Callao at once entered his boat, for he knew that the vessel must bring the new virey of Peru, who was hourly expected. They were all so sure of the deposition of Count Cinchon.

When he arrived on board and was led to the cabin, where the virey was awaiting him, his heart beat faster. But when he had opened the door and beheld Count Cinchon, he stood as if petrified, unable to utter a single word.

"Welcome, Don Rivarez," Cinchon greeted him. "Why do you seem so struck?"

The commandant was now compelled to speak, and he did it the more freely because he was a friend to Cinchon. He had considered Cinchon's cause lost, and it appeared prudent to him to attend to the transmission of the accusing documents from Lima. Cinchon knew this very well, for he had learned it in Spain, but he forgave him on condition that he would not again be guilty of such a wrong.

Rivarez promised this. He was evidently sincerely sorry for what he had done, and Cinchon was mild and friendly as always. Now the commandant opened his heart to the virey.

"You do not know, dear sir," said he, "what has befallen the city of Lima during your absence. "Instead of a beautiful city, you will find a heap of ruins. An earthquake has worked terrible destruction. Many churches, and a great number of houses have fallen and are in ruins, especially in the parts of the city lying near the Rimac."

"How is it with the cathedral and the palace of the virey?" cried Cinchon in horror.

"Strange to say," answered the commandant, "the buildings about the Plazza Major have suffered little or nothing. The distress in the city, however, is indescribable. Many have openly said, that this misfortune has fallen upon them, on account of the great wrong, which they have done to the noble virey."

Here there must be no delay. The virey left Dolores and Hualma in Callao under Huahamac's care and hastened on to Lima.

His friends gave him joyous greeting. His enemies were filled with anxiety and fear. When they saw, however, that he was mild and considerate, they began to count on his forgiveness. He devised wise plans for relief with the assistance of Don Perez, and when Huahamac arrived with those who had been entrusted to his care, he summoned the Indians to aid. Ruins were cleared away, and the building of low houses was at once begun by the order of the virey.

All were full of gratefulness for the noble man, and before the rainy season had set in, Lima had arisen out of its ruins. Nevertheless the fever broke out worse than ever, and the hour had arrived for Huahamac to keep his word.

Hualma accompanied him into the mountains, since Cinchon released her and all other hostages. This confidence which the virey showed the Indians, had a wonderful effect upon the whole nation.

Huahamac called together a council. He gave an account of his voyage across the seas and of the intentions of the Spanish king with respect to the Indians. He promised a happy future, but he made the one condition, that the fever remedy be no longer kept secret from the sufferers.

A murmur of dissent was heard in the circle of the assembly. Now Hualma, in all the attractiveness of her maidenly beauty, clothed after the manner of the women of the Incas, a magnificent crown of feathers on her head, entered the circle.

The effect of her appearance was remarkable. More wonderful still was the effect of her spirited and inspiring address to the people. Overwhelmed by her arguments, they were unbound from their oath by the priests.

A few days later the Indians appeared in the market with the fever bark. The careful use of the remedy saved the lives of almost all those who had been taken sick in Lima, and the dreadful fever was henceforth under control. A blessing was bestowed upon the human family on this and the other side of the sea, which a justifiable hatred had withheld until overcome by Christian love.

As long as Count Cinchon ruled as virey of Peru,

peace continued, and the relation between the Spaniards and the Indians was mutually benficial for a long time to come.

The family of Cinchon and that of Huahamac remained bound together by ties of closest friendship. Their names deserve to be praised among the namens of the benefactors of the human race. But the tree, which provides the healing fever remedy, received Cinchon's name. It is called Cinchona.

www.ingramcontent.com/pod-product-compliance
Lightning Source LLC
Chambersburg PA
CBHW032106080426
42733CB00006B/441